# ASTHMA FREE IN 21 DAYS

# ASTHMA FREE
## IN 21 DAYS

### THE BREAKTHROUGH
### MINDBODY HEALING PROGRAM

Kathryn Shafer, Ph.D., & Fran Greenfield, M.A.

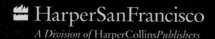 HarperSanFrancisco
*A Division of* HarperCollins*Publishers*

Grateful acknowledgment is made for permission to reprint material copyrighted by the following authors or publishers:

"The Exorcism," "Pine Forest," and "Red Suit" imagery exercises from *Healing Visualizations* by Gerald N. Epstein, M.D. (New York: Bantam Books, 1989). Copyright © 1989 by Gerald N. Epstein, M.D. Reprinted by permission of Bantam Books.

"Autobiography" from *There's a Hole in My Sidewalk* by Portia Nelson (Hillsboro, OR: Beyond Words Publishing, 1993). Copyright © 1989 by Portia Nelson. Reprinted by permission of Beyond Words Publishing.

From "I Can See Clearly Now" by Johnny Nash. Copyright © 1972 by Dovan Music, Inc. All rights reserved. Used by permission of Dovan Music, Inc.

From "Suite Judy Blue Eyes" by Stephen Stills. Copyright © 1969 (Renewed) by Gold Hill Music, Inc. All rights administered by Almo Music Corp. (ASCAP) All rights reserved. Used by permission of Warner Bros. Publications U. S. Inc., Miami, Florida.

ASTHMA FREE IN 21 DAYS: *The Breakthrough Mindbody Healing Program*. Copyright © 2000 by Kathryn Shafer, Ph.D., and Fran Greenfield, M.A. All rights reserved. Printed in the United States of America. No part of this book may be used or reproduced in any manner whatsoever without written permission except in the case of brief quotations embodied in critical articles and reviews. For information address HarperCollins Publishers, Inc., 10 East 53rd Street, New York, NY 10022.

HarperCollins books may be purchased for educational, business, or sales promotional use. For information please write: Special Markets Department, HarperCollins Publishers, Inc., 10 East 53rd Street, New York, NY 10022.

HarperCollins Web site: http://www.harpercollins.com

HarperCollins®, 🅐®, and HarperSanFrancisco™ are trademarks of HarperCollins Publishers, Inc.

FIRST EDITION

*Designed by Lindgren/Fuller Design*

Library of Congress Cataloging-in-Publication Data

Shafer Kathryn.
    Asthma free in 21 days : the breakthrough mindbody healing program / Kathryn Shafer & Fran Greenfield.
    Includes index.
    ISBN 0-06-251597-7 (hc.)
    1. Asthma—Alternative treatment—Popular works.  2. Mind and body—health aspects—Popular works.  I. Greenfield, Fran.  II. Title.

RC591 .S53 2000
616.2'3806—dc21                                       99–056136

00 01 02 03 04 ❖/RRD(H) 10 9 8 7 6 5 4 3 2 1

# CONTENTS

# FOREWORD

by Gerald N. Epstein, M.D.

This book is a tribute to two resolute practitioners of mental imagery and mindbody integration who together have fashioned a masterful, innovative, and successful program for the treatment of asthma based on teaching the patient to heal him- or herself.

The credit for this work goes to Dr. Kathryn Shafer, a doctor of clinical social work who came to see me at the age of thirty-five for the treatment of asthma that had plagued her since the age of fifteen months. After two meetings with me she experienced a healing of the asthmatic condition that has remained stable over the past five years in spite of being exposed to the main triggers usually associated with asthma: upper respiratory infection, allergies (she lives in Florida, one of the worst locations in which asthmatics can live), and emotional conflicts. She experienced all three in profusion and weathered them courageously, and without recurrence. Consequently, she decided to become my student and make her practice the very therapy that she used to heal herself. In doing so she has become a wonderful practitioner helping many people to heal themselves.

The merit for fulfilling the gestation of this book goes to Frances Greenfield, a brilliant practitioner of my work, who has built upon it to create innovative treatment programs for prisoners, alcoholics, and cancer patients, showing them how to heal themselves. Fran used Kathy's story as a springboard, along with Kathy's direct experience and understanding of the asthmatic process, to write this book, which describes the comprehensive mindbody approach that they have tested on their patients with singular success. As in all mindbody therapies, and especially with regard to mental imagery, the patient is empowered and made to be an active participant—the healer in his or her own treatment.

The result of this collaborative effort represents the makings of a breakthrough in the treatment of this devastating disease, currently the leading killer amongst the inner-city population in this country. Asthma has been a riddle for medicine because of the multifaceted dimensions that are so clearly spelled out in the medical literature, yet conventional medical interventions have not significantly stemmed the incidence of this ailment. Also, many patients have been consigned to a state of dependency on the steroids and steroidal inhalants that are frequently prescribed for this condition.

In my breakthrough research in asthma conducted in the mid–1990s under the auspices of the National Institutes of Health, I discovered that by using my mental imagery method, patients were able to stop taking medication altogether, or to substantially reduce it without impairment to their respiratory function. In addition, they were able, in a great majority of cases, to stop using their inhalers.

While my current interests have carried me away from this research, I have felt some measure of gratification that it still lives in the extraordinary development and evolution of that pioneering work, undertaken by these two gifted clinicians. My admiration of them for their fruitful conception and birth of this book is unbounded. Their efforts now open a new door in a new era for a patient-based balanced approach to a psychophysical illness that has eluded the best ministrations that conventional medicine has offered in trying to cure this condition. Kathy and Fran are to be congratulated for bringing—pardon the pun—a breath of fresh air into the treatment of this respiratory malady.

# ACKNOWLEDGMENTS

This book's evolution from a seedling idea to a fully realized manuscript could not have been accomplished without help from the following people.

We wish to thank Doug Abrams, our "miracle editor," who rescued us from oblivion and stretched our talents to the limits. Renee Sedliar, editorial assistant extraordinaire, smoothed the way and helped us bring this project to fruition. Sheryl Gura Rosenberg provided counsel and creativity that were invaluable in developing this manuscript and keeping us on track. Priscilla Stuckey masterminded a brilliant copy-editing job. Lynn Franklin recognized the value of this book and found it a home. And to the special people who shared their personal stories and allowed them to enrich these pages, we are grateful beyond words.

KATHRYN SHAFER AND
FRAN GREENFIELD

I wish to recognize the people who encouraged me to write this book and to live asthma free: Rosalie Shafer, my mother, and Dr. Gerald Epstein, my mentor and friend, who each teach me in a unique way that freedom is loving unconditionally. Hal Shafer, my father, reminds me that acceptance comes from believing in a Higher Power. With Terri Shafer-Villegas, my sister, I share laughter and "FUN." Dorothy Booker is my model of will and leadership. Jacquelyn Dwoskin, whose love encourages me to write and teach. Luba Bozanich, who ran alongside me through the entire 1996 New York City Marathon. My friends who stood by me at the hospital after the accident and inspired me to heal in "record time." Colette Aboulker-Muscat helped me discover my guardian angel and the healing power of the invisible world. Ariel Ford, who had a hunch that my story was worth telling. Candace Rondeaux for all her assistance. And to all the clients and students whose lives merge with mine, I express my gratitude and love.

KATHRYN SHAFER


Beyond the actual writing of a book lies the inspiration and support of many people. In light of this I wish to thank:

My children, Brad and Karen Feinberg, for sharing their strength and loving encouragement. My friends Lauren Adams, Ellie Batt, Phyllis Kahaney, Carol Korbel, Cintra Murchison, and Vry Roussin, who bolstered and supported me from beginning to end. Dr. Gerald Epstein, who has helped me to shape my life and my work. Mary Ann Brussat and Viviane Lind for their wise counsel. John Schuler for giving generously of his time and talent. Noelle Bikoff for her graphics. Russell Mason for his eleventh-hour editorial contribution. My sister, Harriet Surace, for her unwavering belief in me. Harold Herbstman, whose love sustains me always. And my parents, Betty and Sam Greenfield, for their extraordinary grace, and for giving me the gift of life.

FRAN GREENFIELD

# INTRODUCTION

*Fear is the lock, and laughter the key to your heart.*
CROSBY, STILLS AND NASH,
"SUITE JUDY BLUE EYES"

Without breath, life is impossible. With limited breath, it's exhausting and frightening. Yet every day more than seventeen million Americans, almost five million of these children, along with millions of other asthmatics throughout the world, struggle to breathe freely.[1] This natural function of breathing in and breathing out is one that most people take for granted. But for asthma sufferers, too often it's a complex, mystifying, and unnerving event.

The disease we call asthma knows no boundaries. It affects people from all walks of life. They come from rural areas, small towns and large cities, all climates and cultures. No two are identical. But the one thing they have in common—attacks of asthma that leave them gasping for breath—binds them together in an immediate and meaningful way.

No longer is this illness an oddity. Asthma ranks sixth out of all diseases as the cause for hospitalization and first in hospital admissions and emergency room visits for children. It invades the lives of the young, the middle-aged, and the elderly; male and female; all racial groups; and every social and economic segment of the population. More than one billion dollars are spent annually on this complicated, life-threatening illness. And day by day its threat increases.

Until recently asthmatics depended on conventional Western medicine for treatment. Yet despite decades of research, the medical model can offer only temporary relief and no real solution. To preclude and suppress symptoms, it advocates the use of bronchodilators, steroids, preventive aids, and pulmonary devices. But little interest has been expressed in natural alternatives, which it considers unproven and ineffective. The light at the end of the tunnel has been obscured by this limited point of view, one that encourages the patient to take a submissive role in the healing process. Such an outlook neglects the premise that asthmatics can do a great deal more than medicate themselves to lessen the severity and the frequency of their attacks.

It is not surprising that asthmatics, who in the past saw themselves as victims, have begun turning to "alternative" approaches.[2] Our current health care system, based on the authoritarian model of expert and patient, has relentlessly furthered a victim mentality. This results in a sense of helplessness and even embarrassment. In plain words, asthmatics are taught to believe that they should:

1. Hand over all important health care decisions to those "experts" who are medically knowledgeable
2. Depend on prescribed medications to prevent, address, and suppress symptoms
3. Admit no responsibility *for* or meaningful relationship *to* their illness
4. Regard anything other than allopathic medicine as suspect and/or unreliable
5. Be compliant patients and accept asthma as a life sentence

The burgeoning interest in natural remedies and mindbody medicine has generated a new model of healing, one that encourages responsibility for our own well-being and fosters an awareness of the true meaning of health and healing. Health means more than freedom from symptoms of disease. It means being whole. While *curing* may remove physical symptoms, it provides only superficial relief, leaving the roots of disease untouched. But *healing* goes much deeper. It involves the integration of mind and body—a unification so seamless we have deleted the usual hyphen from the word *mindbody* throughout the book to reflect its true meaning.

This is essentially different from the conventional medical viewpoint, which sees the body as a machine, focuses on what's wrong with it, and then tries to fix it as quickly as possible. Instead, this process turns you toward the illness and encourages listening nonjudgmentally to what it may be telling you.

No doubt conventional medicine makes a valuable contribution to our lives, particularly in emergency situations. However, routinely prescribing inhalers, bronchodilators, and steroids creates dependency and does not substantially alter the disease or get to its source. Asthma, which has been challenging medical science for hundreds of years, has yet to be looked at as anything more than a dangerous and discomforting symptom, or addressed through a whole-person, mindbody vision. Although some experts do admit the role of psychological stress in triggering and exacerbating asthma symptoms, the mind has only barely been tapped as a method for prevention, symptom relief, and healing.

In contrast, mindbody medicine addresses not only our physical symptoms but our emotional suffering as well. To make the power of the mind available for healing, *Asthma Free in 21 Days* introduces a system called the FUN Program. Using the acronym FUN may surprise some readers. But we have thoughtfully chosen it as the core, healing stance of this program and have used it successfully with our clients in private practice and in workshops throughout the country. FUN, a quality too often missing in the lives of asthmatics, far from trivializes asthma. It is, in fact, an *antidote* to the constriction and seriousness of asthma's symptoms. FUN stands for *Focus, Undo,* and *Now Act,* each segment of which is discussed and demonstrated throughout the book.

Recent research by Dr. Lee Burk, a neurologist at Loma Linda University in California, has definitively shown the positive effect of laughter, joy, and fun on our immune response and physiology.

Burk, whose work in the field of psychoneuroimmunology, the scientific study of how emotions are related to immune function, is widely published, and calls *mirthfulness* the "frontier of frontiers." Clearly, even the bastions of medical science have begun to acknowledge what we propose in this book: that there is an intimate relationship of body and mind, of emotion and health. And that "having fun" embodies a genuine healing effect in our lives.

The FUN program provides the growing population of asthmatics with a mindbody healing system that is effective and safe. With the permission of our clients who have participated in this work, their personal stories have been included. Emily, the nine-year-old child; Bob, the law student; Linda, the therapist—each wanted to gain freedom from the fears and restrictions that asthma imposed, and it was through this work that each became able to live an active, joyful, revitalized life.

By seeing the asthma from an emotional, social, and spiritual perspective, asthmatics begin to lay the groundwork for living freely and authentically. This is a process that goes beyond temporary, mechanical symptom reduction. Instead, it helps you to discover the symptom's meaning and to make sense of the suffering that had previously seemed random and painful. Once engaged in this new stance, you become able to shine a powerful light into the darkness. And what seemed to be only wishful thinking—such as reducing or dispensing with medications and living a more spontaneous life—is suddenly possible.

The program and techniques we present here allow asthmatics to make an amazing turn. After much pain and frustration with asthma, children as young as six as well as people in their senior years have learned to use a repertoire of simple tools for creating a better quality of life, not just for themselves but for their families as well. The benefits you enjoy once you begin to use this program include significant relief from physical symptoms; freedom from old habits and limited thinking; higher energy levels; overall health improvement; and joy in living. It can take *less than two minutes* to notice a change, and once this change has begun it becomes fulfilling in ways that go far beyond the asthma. Relationships, energy, and productivity are affected. Anxiety, fatigue, and depression are transformed as well. And as long as the work is maintained in your everyday life, the transformation remains lasting and powerful.

Our message is simple: you can become your own authority. This involves being willing to trade unconsciousness for awareness, subservience for autonomy, slavery for freedom. No disease process, prognosis, or limitation is carved in stone; neither is the game plan that you use to address it. This does not mean that you should throw away your medications and disregard your doctor's advice. However, it does mean that there is no "right" or "wrong" way to deal with asthma, only *your own way*. When you allow the asthma to speak to you, it can serve as your compass. This compass can lead you toward a place within yourself that holds the information and wisdom for creating an effective recovery plan and beginning to live an asthma-free life.

## WHO CAN BENEFIT FROM THIS BOOK?

Many people may find this program useful: adults and children with asthma, relatives and friends of asthmatics, and all health care professionals who are interested in a more open, creative approach for their clients, patients, and/or for themselves. This work is meant to be shared. Although the program was originally developed for asthmatics, those who suffer from other disorders and difficulties can make excellent use of it as well.

## HOW TO USE THIS BOOK

Just as there is no "right" way to deal with asthma, there is no "right" way to read this book or to follow this program. How you approach it is up to you. Do the exercises in the order they appear in the text, or return to them after you have gotten an overall feel for the program. Underline passages that interest you, or write notes in the margins as you go along. Whether you have just been diagnosed with asthma or have had it for years, you start by committing to the program for the next 21 days. During this time, pay attention to the changes that occur (large or small, emotional or physical) in your health and your daily life. Healing isn't static; it's an ongoing process. So if you like what you see, follow up your initial commitment with additional cycles and a consistent practice of the work to maintain its beneficial effects.

The exercises throughout the book address asthma in several ways, and the benefits you receive are both short and long term. Some exercises elicit immediate relief of symptoms. Others bring about a deeper healing by expanding your awareness and allowing you to see the asthma in relationship to your life as a whole. Any of these may become part of your healing plan. Those used for immediate symptom relief will be marked by this symbol: ✳ Yet the system is flexible. While some exercises may be designated for deeper healing and awareness, they often provide immediate relief as well. If this occurs, make a note of it.

Many healing processes have been included in this book, but there's no need to overwhelm yourself by trying to do them all at once. For one person, a daily practice might involve doing only one exercise, while another person might use four or five. Many people like to increase the number of exercises as they go along until they find what feels right for them. In most instances, we advise you to use the imagery exercises for 21 days. This is no arbitrary number. In many traditions it is viewed as the amount of time it takes to break a habit. If the symptom, habit, or disorder has not disappeared after 21 days, additional cycles may be added. If you are satisfied before the 21 days, you may stop a particular exercise sooner, though we recommend completing the whole cycle.

Every practice or exercise in the book has proven valuable, yet the only way to experience this work is to actually use it. Quite simply, what you get out of the program will be in direct proportion to what you put in. In this respect, mind medicine is not so different from regular medicine: when you follow the prescription as advised you are far more likely to get the results you're looking for.

## WHAT'S INCLUDED

In chapter 1, Kathy shares her personal story from the time she was diagnosed with asthma at the age of fifteen months until she defied the odds and crossed the finish line of the New York City Marathon in 1996.

Chapter 2 presents an overview of asthma including: a simple definition of asthma; a discussion of who is at risk; its triggers and effects; and a brief description of the kinds of treatment available. It informs you of the differences between conventional and non-conventional medicine and provides a description of *mind medicine*, particularly of mental imagery.

Chapter 3 sets the stage for creating a new relationship with asthma. It shows how to pay attention to your personal experience with this disease, and it includes a mindbody questionnaire. This questionnaire gives you a chance to discover life-enhancing information about making changes that will allow you to breathe freely and fully.

Chapter 4 introduces the process of mental imagery, a technique and a stance, that is both practical and healing. You'll learn about its history, along with recent research on mental imagery, including the Lenox Hill study run by Dr. Gerald Epstein, which showed a stunning 47 percent improvement in pulmonary capacity of the participants using mental imagery. You will also begin to experience the benefits of imagery; you'll learn how to start doing it on your own; and you'll find examples of how imagery can be used as a comprehensive tool for healing. The exercises here and throughout the book work quickly, some in less than two minutes. As the title states, in the 21 days it takes to complete them, you can actually become asthma free. In addition, this chapter introduces you to the *Committee,* those false selves who sabotage your progress while at the same time insisting that without their advice you could not possibly survive.

Chapter 5 introduces FUN, the healing stance that is the heart of this program. FUN is powerful mind medicine. It emphasizes the importance of joy as the core emotional element for healing asthma. It teaches you how to Focus, Undo, and Now Act in your own healing interests. When you expand your awareness regarding asthma with the FUN techniques, you begin to recognize the beliefs and emotions that feed its roots. It's at this point you can choose to reverse your symptoms. Having fun is never frivolous or unnecessary if you want to heal; it's actually essential to living asthma free.

Chapter 6 introduces the process of *Focusing,* the first part of the FUN program. Focusing is a process of expanding your awareness and becoming conscious of your thoughts, beliefs, attitudes, and actions. This is done without judging or being attached. You observe and listen to asthma symptoms as valuable indicators. The mindbody connection is demonstrated through exercises and techniques that bypass the logical, judgmental mind. Focusing is the first step in the process of paying attention, which is an absolute necessity for genuine healing.

Chapter 7 describes and demonstrates the process of *Undoing,* the second part of FUN. Undoing goes far beyond coping strategies. It shows you how to reverse illness and difficulty; how to Undo past traumas through imagery, and how to vanquish symptoms by using a newly researched writing technique. Here the emphasis is on Undoing those core beliefs that make asthmatics feel separate and limited. Through special exercises and the shared experiences of others, this popular myth of abnormality and limitation is put to rest.

Chapter 8 illustrates how you may *Now Act* to seize the moment and transform the program into a lived, active experience. We provide you with techniques that motivate action—not just any action but the kind that generates healing. This chapter demonstrates how Now Acting in meaningful ways allows you to enter more fully into the present instead of living falsely in the future or the past. This, along with a perspective of nonattachment to the outcome, helps you to leave behind the pain of your old story while beginning to live and breathe freely in the here and now.

Chapter 9 presents research on childhood asthma, along with experiences of children and parents dealing with this disease in their everyday lives. Examples and suggestions show how kids can use the FUN approach to help themselves do more than just reach for medication. One particularly moving story tells of Emily, a nine-year-old girl who made her own personal journey of recovery using the techniques shared in this book.

Chapter 10 gives kids a chance to "do their own thing" by providing them with a special "FUN Guide for Kids." Exercises designed especially for children will show them how to create their own imagery, which adults can do too.

Chapter 11 offers a unique mindbody perspective regarding three important concerns: exercise-induced asthma, nutrition, and environment. This expanded mindbody view opens new possibilities and options. For the first time, the various types of asthma are presented here in relationship to your entire life experience instead of being seen as automatic triggers.

Chapter 12 presents you with three 21-day healing plans that are flexible and comprehensive: one general plan for adults, a second for those with exercise-induced asthma, and a third for kids. You may choose to follow any of these just as they are, customize them for yourself, or take on the responsibility of creating a plan on your own. The Complete Index of Exercises, also contained here, helps you to do just this. All these plans are a form of self-care that designates *you* as the primary care provider. They afford you a practical process for living asthma free.

The essential tool for healing is *listening*—with both the heart and the mind. Listening to your symptoms is a way of listening to yourself. When you cease to analyze and judge what goes on in life, you can suspend the habits of blaming, comparing, or complaining, and you can instead create a space between you and your difficulties. Releasing these mental habits expands your awareness and cultivates a healthier outlook. Once you take responsibility in this way you may quite naturally generate a healing that is far deeper than you have ever thought possible.

We encourage you to use this new perspective as a way to trust yourself and your natural sense of what you want and need. When you are your own authority, the approval of others becomes far less important. You begin to live life as who you really are—acknowledging your body as your fundamental truth and your symptoms as its messages. When you listen to it openly, you will be moved and surprised by how much it knows.

# CHAPTER 1

# FROM VICTIM
# TO VICTOR

*I can see clearly now the rain is gone;*
*I can see all obstacles in my way;*
*Gone are the dark clouds that had me blind;*
*It's gonna be a bright, bright sunshiny day.*
    JOHNNY NASH, "I CAN SEE CLEARLY NOW"

November 6, 1996. It is the morning of the New York City Marathon. I wake while it is still dark. To protect myself from the unseasonable early autumn cold, I dress in several layers of running gear. Suddenly, moments from my past come flooding back. It's then and now all at once.

*I am five, crying because I want to play outside with the other kids, and my mother forbids it. I am sixteen, sneaking away from my friends to take my medication. I am twenty-five, angry because I can't run without carrying my inhaler. Then suddenly, it's last night. I am watching them paint the finish line in a wide, red swath across the black pavement of Central Park. The lights of the city begin coming on in the surrounding buildings. I have a hard time believing I'm finally here.*

I exhale and come back to now, to this minute, this second, to the sound of Sting on the radio. For a few moments I sit there with the music, just inhaling the sound. Then I close my eyes and imagine doing what I've been told my whole life was impossible: I see myself crossing the finish line triumphant, breathing freely, completing the race that for years I've hoped and prayed I would one day be able to run.

My goal is simple: to run through all five boroughs of my favorite city, to have fun, to complete the race, and not to get caught up in the competition. How well I do, how long it takes, isn't important. Just running this marathon and completing it is enough!

At 10:45 A.M., twenty-nine thousand runners wait to begin. The sunlight glints off the Verrazano Narrows Bridge, and I feel an excitement so electric my body vibrates. At the sound of the starting gun, we begin the race. Through the noise of the helicopters overhead, I hear the voices of the crowds on the opposite shore, the pulsating music, and words shouted in more languages than I can count.

As I run I sense changes in the pavement beneath my feet, in the neighborhoods, the odors, the play of shadows and light, and at this moment, life is perfect. I am exactly where I want to be, doing what I have dreamed of doing for years.

*The doctor's words stun me. "You will never run a marathon," he says. I ask more questions. I argue. He shrugs, looks at his watch, and reminds me that I am lucky to be alive. I have never forgotten his voice. Wish he could see me now.*

I remind myself to go easy. After ten miles my right leg, the one I fractured during a nearly fatal accident two years ago, begins to hurt. I concentrate on maintaining my own steady rhythm. I imagine breathing in the blue line painted along the course, the same blue line I visited the day before; somehow this eases my pain and carries me forward.

Thirteen point one miles. I'm halfway there. The summit of the Pulaski Bridge is quiet, suspended in time, with the towers of Manhattan looming beyond.

Fifteen miles. We approach the 59th Street Bridge. Thousands of us pound across the grating toward Manhattan, where crowds line the streets. They hand us chocolate, apples, and oranges that we reach out and grab. At 83rd Street and First Avenue, my sister waits for me, along with some friends. They smile and shout out my name; they are relieved that I'm still going strong. I use their encouragement as a talisman of hope.

*My sister is playing outside with her friends. She is younger, but she can do things I can't. I am jealous. I wish for some kind of magic to set me free. I wait months, years. But the magic words never get spoken. The spell remains intact. I pray. I promise. I bargain. I dream.*

Twenty miles. We enter the Bronx. The discomfort in my leg is intense, but I force myself to keep moving. I pass Yankee Stadium. I get a rush remembering their World Series victory. I begin to sing "I Can See Clearly Now," a Johnny Nash song I heard while driving to work a few months ago. It reminds me of the long journey I have taken to get here. Other runners join in. I feel energized and inspired.

We enter Harlem. I've been running five hours. The enthusiasm of the crowd pulls me along. It helps to keep the tiredness at bay. Not so long now, I think.

Five miles left. I begin to anticipate what they call the "dreaded hills" of Central Park. It seems only moments later that I see the Metropolitan Museum on 82nd Street and realize by some miracle we have passed them.

Toward 59th Street, the crowds thin out. As we enter the park, those still waiting outside the Plaza Hotel cheer us on as a pathway shaped by the late afternoon sun guides me to the finish line. Crossing it in slow motion, I wrap my mind around this moment, this feeling, this lifetime dream.

I am runner 26,948, woman 6,806, a *champion!* Without medication and suffering no ill consequences, I have completed one of the world's most famous marathons—*me*, an asthmatic since early childhood.

*The spell is broken. The magic is real, and I want it to last forever.*

## AGAINST ALL ODDS

This is light-years from where I began. Diagnosed with asthma when I was fifteen months old, I spent much of my early life in pediatric hospital rooms, under oxygen tents, and taking frequent doses of medications. Even when I was home, business continued as usual (medical business that is), with me paying weekly visits to asthma specialists who prescribed daily doses of inhalants, allergy shots, and oral medicines. I can still recall waiting long hours for doctors to give me shots and scratch tests while being constantly warned about the dangers of asthma.

My mother and I became accustomed to this fragmented, unnatural world of medicines, painful treatments, restricted living, and fear. I had been thoroughly indoctrinated into accepting this way of life and the rules I needed to obey in order to survive. But a part of me rebelled. I was a child. I wanted to play outside with my friends. Despite my desire to be the same as the others, I knew I was different. They played without wheezing and losing their breath, something I had never done. Instead, I was confined to a room that resembled an oversized oxygen tent, with plastic curtains on the windows, a gray linoleum floor, and a special respiratory apparatus installed near my ugly, adjustable, hospital bed.

I submitted to my medical regimen without much complaint, taking whatever the doctors prescribed. I was afraid of breaking the rules, since any slipup might leave me unable to breathe. What a tremendous burden this was! No matter how I figured, it never made sense. When I asked my doctors if I would ever be well, able to run and play, they told me I had a "serious medical problem." "You were born with asthma, and it will always be with you. Just get used to it," they said.

As I grew older, the asthma worsened and my medications and therapies became more extreme. By the time I was seven I was, for all practical purposes, barricaded in my sterile room, taking oral medication every four hours, and dedicating another two hours a day to inhalation therapy. Under my mother's supervision, I inhaled a mixture of medicines from the pulmonary pump near my bed. I would imagine this machine was a monster and would fantasize kicking it over to free myself. But my fear of not being able to breathe kept me totally compliant, hating the therapies and medications yet feeling indebted to them for my daily existence.

Another part of my therapy involved my mother pounding my back and chest to loosen the mucus that accumulated in my bronchial tubes. Each time she arrived at my bedroom door, I cringed. I knew what was coming. Despite any comfort she might give me, her arrival meant the pain of another treatment. Much later I would finally realize how deeply this had affected me—how intricately woven together pain, nurturing, love, and the effort of staying alive had become. It's not surprising that this peculiar pattern would determine the nature of my relationships in the future. For me, love and pain were now intimately associated.

## REVERSING MY LIFE SENTENCE

Even though the doctors offered no hope, a small part of me refused to accept their gloominess. I became determined to reverse this life sentence of limitation and dependency. Being out of school so much gave me extra time to read and study. I wanted to be like the others, to be good at something, and my schoolwork seemed to be the answer. My success with academics nurtured my confidence. I had found a way to excel, and I used this as a starting point. By seventh grade I began to spread my wings. Not exactly flying, but finally starting to get off the ground, I stopped waiting to be cured; instead I began to *act as if* I were normal. Sure, I had to carry my medication around with me all the time, but I hid it away and took it as both the doctor and my mother ordered, sneaking into the girls' room to do it when no one was around.

By this time my natural interest in sports began to blossom. Softball and track were my favorites: of course my mother warned me to be careful and insisted on picking me up after practice, but I refused. I wanted to be normal, and sports made me feel that way, far more than the honors in academics. Instead of worrying about my illness, I placed my attention on doing what I loved. I had spent enough of my life hidden away in my room. I wanted and needed to break free, to be part of the group. Sports seemed to be the answer, and I used every ounce of will I had to keep the asthma from limiting me.

But my good intentions were often ambushed by my driving need to be like the others. As a teenager, I gave my body mixed messages. On the one hand, I longed to be well, to breathe freely, while on the other, I chose to smoke cigarettes with my friends. The smoking made me one of "them." It eased the embarrassment of dealing with my illness. I knew the smoking was counterproductive, even life threatening, yet I wanted to fit in so desperately that I was willing to ignore the possible consequences.

While I realized that trying to find out *why* I had asthma was futile and self-victimizing, exploring the mental and emotional issues of my illness provoked my interest. In college I studied social work, hoping to discover a link between the emotional and psychological elements of physical illness. In the back of my mind there was always a need to find out more about asthma and ultimately to use what I found to educate and heal others as well as myself. Through my studies it became clear that emotional upset and stress often coincided with the onset of asthmatic attacks, and in my own life I couldn't help but notice how an attack would come on when I was emotionally distressed.

Gradually, this relationship between emotional and mental stress and the onset of asthmatic symptoms became the focal point of my interests. And though I continued to be what the medical profession calls a "compliant" patient, taking my medications as ordered, I wondered whether this was the wisest, most effective approach. Always on the lookout for nonconventional treatments, my hope was that one day I would be done with all medications, able to breathe easily and to run without carrying inhalers.

## THE TURNING POINT

After a ten-year search I heard of a book called *Healing Visualizations* by Dr. Gerald Epstein, a psychiatrist in New York City, who had developed a healing practice called mental imagery based on the teachings first elucidated by the biblical prophets. From what I had read, these brief exercises worked very well with both emotional and physical illnesses, including asthma. At first I was skeptical. How could a few minutes each day of a simple mental technique cure me when the best doctors had failed? As for the biblical prophets, I had more than a little difficulty relating them to the actual healing of asthma. My defense system went into red alert. Every belief I had secretly harbored regarding the well-known limitations of this illness, its serious nature, and its resistance to healing became instant ammunition to shoot down this possibility.

But I had tried everything else. The list seemed endless, exhausting, and expensive: conventional medication, group therapy, individual counseling, psychiatry, bioenergetics, homeopathy, aromatherapy, massage, meditation, rebirthing, nutritional changes, exercise, and smoking cessation. And though most of these had helped for brief periods of time, none had offered the kind of deep, lasting changes for which I had been searching.

### My First Imagery Experience
Putting my reservations aside, I called and made an appointment with Dr. Epstein. He inquired about my medical history and then asked me if I really wanted to heal the asthma—a strange question to ask an asthmatic. But as he already knew (and as I was coming to understand), serious emotional currents run through every

illness. Often this involves a deep conflict or ambivalence that eventually manifests as a symptom. When I affirmed wholeheartedly that yes, I wanted to do this, he told me that he would give me an imagery exercise that I needed to practice regularly without discussing it with anyone else. When I asked for reassurance that this would work, he simply suggested that I do it and see what happens. Unlike my medical doctors, he would make no predictions.

After some brief preparation for imaging, he gave me an exercise that was nothing like what I expected. Instead of using anatomical images of my organs—specifically the difficulty with my lungs—Dr. Epstein guided me through an exercise that required me to reveal the face of the person whose presence and influence was restricting my breathing and limiting my life. When the first face I saw was my mother's, I was shocked. After all, this was someone I loved, the person who had been so good to me! I was then directed to remove this person from my body while saying in my imagination that she was no longer welcome there and would never be allowed to enter it again. Despite the tears that ran down my face, I managed to remove her. The next face that appeared was of the man who had been my boyfriend for the last seven years. Again I felt uncomfortable, and I resisted. But I already knew that something had to be done about the relationship, that it couldn't stay as it was. Though all this was painful, I sensed that by imaginally removing these people, I was finally separating from them and releasing myself from their influence—the kind of influence that prevented me from breathing freely.

Immediately I knew this work was different from anything I had ever done before. There were no set limits in my imagination, no stories about the future or regrets about the past to get in my way. This was the beginning of my healing process, the moment when I reached a turning point and chose to take the path of truth, no matter how uncomfortable it made me. Through employing the technique of imagery I had entered what I would soon learn to call the invisible world and had brought back with me a revelation that was to change the course of my life. Yet after so many false starts I wasn't sure that I could trust it. Despite this skepticism, I decided to do the work—to experiment with it and to wait and see.

For the next 21 days (which is the time it takes to break a habit) I practiced the exercise faithfully. Immediately I started to feel different. By the end of the first cycle I was off all oral medication (Theodur and Prednisone) and down to one inhaler (Proventil). All this within a month! Through using this simple technique, the door to genuine healing had begun to open. At last I had found an effective process that was simple and direct and that harbored no ill side effects.

If anyone had told me beforehand that this would happen, I wouldn't have believed it. How could this technique, which took so little time, produce such powerful results? But the physical changes were undeniable. So I decided to continue the work with the intention of finally dispensing with my inhaler. This was a giant step for me. Over the years I had formed a strong attachment to this device, actually fearing that without immediate access to it I might die. But with another exercise—one that allowed me to substitute the image of removing a weight from my chest whenever breathing became difficult, I was able to replace the squirt of my inhaler with a new kind of prescription, a dose of imagery. And though initially I kept the inhaler with me, eventually I found I could leave it behind, even when I ran, something I never thought I would be able to do.


## CHOOSING LIFE

Through doing this work I have come to believe there is a *core question* for each of us, one we need to answer if we want to live a whole life. Six months later, when Dr. Epstein asked me if I wanted to live, I knew I had encountered mine. The shock of his question unnerved me. An honest answer would reveal the secret I had been so ashamed to admit, but there was no turning back. Even though I knew what I was about to say might affect everything and everyone close to me, I admitted that I wanted to die. As the words came out of my mouth, instantly a giant weight was lifted off my chest. Where before there had been heaviness and gloom, for the first time in my life there was a sense of possibility, of release and exhilaration.

For years I had been in the habit of giving myself mixed messages, some saying "live," others "die." It was not that I consciously put it in such unsubtle terms. It was far more covert, played out through self-sabotage, indecision, and an unwillingness to release what was familiar even if I felt like it was killing me. You know the saying "I'll do this even if it kills me"? I had become a master of just that kind of thinking. Once I uttered the words "I want to die," it was clear that I had to make a decision to let go of the past and of my life as I currently knew it. This meant seeing each moment as valuable, irreplaceable. It included acknowledging that I am in relationship with all that goes on in my life even when I am in pain, even when life isn't the way I think it's supposed to be. In my heart, I knew that making the conscious choice to live was a commitment to seek the healing power that could be found only inside myself.

It was at this point I began to sense that in some way what happens to me isn't random, chaotic, and meaningless; it is born of my beliefs, thoughts, feelings, and actions. This stance of personal responsibility for my every thought and action was new to me and somewhat uncomfortable at first. Though I felt it was true, it was something I had yet to understand. The concept of even the most difficult events in life having value, meaning, and purpose was virtually the opposite of what I had been taught. But it gave me hope to think that this shift in my thinking could change my life and how I lived it, making even painful experiences things from which I could learn.

In August of 1994, a car driven by a drunk driver almost killed me while I was training for the New York City Marathon. Hit from behind, I flipped up onto the hood, where I hit the windshield and was thrown fifty feet, landing in some shrubbery at the side of the road. Fortunately, an off-duty paramedic stopped to help me and immediately called 911. I was flown by trauma-hawk to St. Mary's Trauma Center, where my injuries were diagnosed as a compound fracture of my right leg, lacerations and a concussion to the back of my head, and severe lacerations of my face and ear. Plastic, neuro-, and orthopedic surgeons were called in immediately. They inserted a rod in my right leg through the knee and down to my ankle, which was held in place with nuts and bolts, and my face, ear, and the back of my head were repaired. It wasn't until later, when I became conscious and complained about pain in my right shoulder, that they discovered it was fractured as well. In addition, the concussion I had sustained was severe enough that I had difficulty recalling what was happening from one moment to the next.

With no guarantee that I would walk, let alone run again, I participated in my recovery, using intense physical therapy, along with my new outlook on life and imagery prescriptions to ensure my healing. My perspective on the accident, based on the concept of value, meaning, and purpose that I described above, made me realize that I was not a victim. I knew in a way that I could not yet explain that this experience was related to my deep need to *break* with the parts of my life that had kept me from moving on. This by no means indicates that I purposely caused this accident to happen. But it does reveal a stunning relationship between my mental and emotional state and the physical event itself. Again, this perspective does not avow that my beliefs and thoughts *caused* the car to hit me or caused me to place myself in harm's way. Yet I knew that this incident could teach me something about myself and my life: it was now my job to determine what that something might be. I recall lying in bed thinking:

*I'm going to be here for a while. So how do I want to use this time? I can lie here feeling depressed and sorry for myself, or I can turn this around and transform my pain into something useful.*

It was at this moment of awakening that I decided to share this way of thinking and healing. I wanted to give others an opportunity to see life's challenges from this new perspective. My pain and discomfort held value, and in my journal I began to keep track of my emotional and physical progress.

In terms of practical methods, my program included the daily practice of mental imagery that involved seeing the actual healing of my bones,[1] creating a prayer collage (a technique described in chapter 8) to provide me with a concrete, visual stimulus for seeing myself fully recovered, and using music as a way of engaging my body in the will to live.

Despite the trauma of this experience, within three months of the accident I returned to work in a wheelchair, never having suffered an asthma attack. Within four months, I completed my dissertation and walked onstage to receive my diploma. My last surgery was in December of 1995. By February of 1996, I began to train for the marathon. I wanted to run again, to get back to feeling "myself." But I wasn't the same. In choosing life, I had chosen change. And by deciding that neither the accident nor the asthma would hold me back—that I would run in the next New York City Marathon—I had embarked on a path that would take me in a completely different direction from where I had been before. This new direction affected my professional life as well. The way I worked with my clients took a tremendous turn. Instead of acting as an authority (having a doctor-patient relationship with them), I chose to be an educator—to teach people how to become their *own* authorities and to find value and meaning in the difficulties of life, even in the chronic pain and fear associated with asthma.

The following two chapters give you an overview of both the conventional, medical approach to asthma and of the mindbody method that changed my life, as well as the lives of many other asthmatics who have found deeper healing than they ever thought possible.

CHAPTER 2

# MEET
# THE MONSTER

## Exploring Your
## Relationship with Asthma

*Acceptance without proof is the fundamental characteristic of Western religion. Rejection without proof is the fundamental characteristic of Western science.*

GARY ZUKOV

This chapter shares information about asthma that may seem basic, but we strongly suggest that you at least skim through, since you may find, as we do, that something valuable can often be discovered amid the familiar. To ease the way, we have kept this chapter concise, clear, and devoid of confusing or unfamiliar medical terminology. What you will find is a definition of asthma; an overview of the conventional and nonconventional medical perspectives; an important clarification of the essential differences between the two types of medicine; and a summary of both allopathic and natural mindbody therapies currently available for treating asthma.

## WHAT IS ASTHMA?

Asthma is one of the most common diseases of modern times and accounts for more absences from work and school than any other chronic illness. It is the leading cause of visits to doctors' offices and often results in emergency room visits, hospitalization during severe attacks, and sometimes death. To gain a comprehensive understanding of this disease, it's important to acknowledge that asthma is more than just a physical ailment. It is a complex *psychophysiological* (or mental, emotional, and physical) disorder in which the airways are supersensitive to a number of stimuli. With asthma, for reasons conventional medicine is not able to understand, this sensitivity triggers the immune system to become chronically overactive and to go on the offensive unnecessarily. This leads to inflammation, which generates a narrowing of the bronchi, the branching tubes leading into the lungs. This narrowing is called bronchoconstriction or bronchospasm, and it results in impaired breathing. In response to the inflammation, the bronchial tubes begin to secrete mucus. This causes obstruction of the bronchi and their smallest parts, the bronchioles. "I feel like I'm breathing through a straw" is how asthmatics commonly describe this experience.

Whatever the so-called causes and triggers may be, the physiological response is the same—a chronic inflammation, narrowed bronchial passages, particularly when breathing out, and a feeling of being smothered. Once labored breathing begins, people often react by becoming anxious, even panicked. In turn, this tightens musculature, restricts airflow further, and increases the discomfort even more, creating a downward spiral of physical and emotional distress.

Often we hear asthma referred to as a chronic disease because attacks may recur repeatedly year after year, yet asthma has been known to disappear gradually during childhood, and it can be reversed at any time during its course.[1] Asthmatics vary in the severity of their symptoms and in their responses. They also vary in how they deal with the illness as part of their lives. Since the illness is elusive and its symptoms are broad, asthma has been baffling science for centuries. Yet many conventional and nonconventional practitioners believe a lot can be done to control asthma—and that with a combination of self-care and professional treatment most asthmatics can lead normal, healthy, active lives.

## WHO HAS ASTHMA?

People of all ages in all parts of the world have this disease, and it surfaces most often in childhood. Both sexes are at risk, but over a third of the cases are found in children under the age of eighteen. Certain ethnic groups appear more vulnerable than others. For instance, African Americans have a 50 percent higher rate of severe asthma than the rest of the population and are hospitalized for it far more often than whites. Native Americans also have a comparatively high number of asthmatics among them.

## THE SIGNS AND SYMPTOMS

Asthma often manifests as tightness in the chest, coughing, difficulty inhaling and exhaling (particularly the latter), and wheezing. But these symptoms do not all necessarily appear together or in every case. During an attack the parts of the lung most directly affected are the bronchi and bronchioles, those tubes that facilitate the passage of oxygen into the body and through which carbon dioxide is expelled.

An asthma attack can be brief, lasting for several minutes, or it may last as long as several days. A severe, prolonged attack can be life threatening, requiring special treatment such as inhalation therapy or the use of oxygen and even hospitalization. These

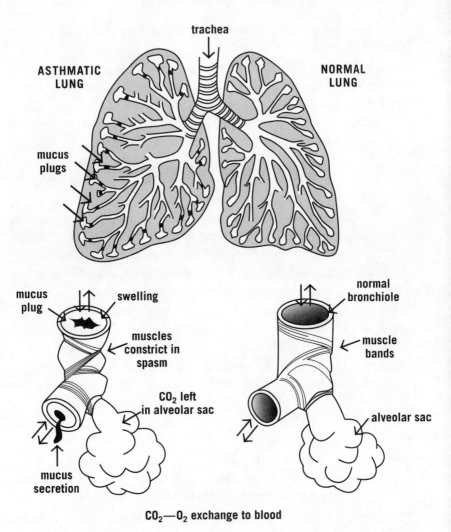

*Figure 2.1*

measures generally last only as long as the attack. Asthma is not known to cause serious damage to the heart or lungs. However, severe asthma can lead to secondary health problems if not properly addressed.

# WHAT TRIGGERS THIS BREATH-TAKING DISEASE?

Asthma can begin at any age, and it may be triggered by a multitude of things, either alone or in combination, varying from one person to the next. It often starts with a virus, an allergic reaction, or a cold. The dramatic rise in the number of asthmatics in recent years has been something of a mystery. One popular premise suggests that our current emphasis on suppressing childhood diseases through medications like antibiotics, vaccines, and so forth is causing this increase. Instead of the immune system developing its natural function of learning to fight off infection, it becomes dependent on these outside interventions. Thus by not allowing the immune system to gather strength and maturity, we inadvertently but actively have disabled it.

Unfortunately, though the early use of medical intervention may have helped us escape the inconvenience and fear of dealing with normal childhood disease, our so-called victory has left us more vulnerable than ever to the allergens, bacteria, and viruses that are natural players in our environment. By avoiding part of our normal experience and labeling it "bad," our immune systems have become weaker, not stronger, while the allergens, viruses, and bacteria have turned the tables on us by becoming stronger and less vulnerable.

## Allergies

Not all people with allergies have asthma, and not all asthmatics are allergic. When you are prone to allergies, the immune system becomes sensitized to one or several substances called allergens and overreacts to these with an inflammatory response. Common allergens include mold spores, pollen, house dust, cockroaches, dust mites, animal dander, cigarette smoke, or certain foods such as orange juice and dairy products. Geography also plays a role: inner city residents (people in poor urban neighborhoods) are exposed to a protein in cockroach feces that acts as an antigen and can trigger attacks. Coastal residents are more susceptible to dust mites, whose feces become allergens once they are airborne. And in southern coastal regions, such as Florida, mold spores and humidity are often a problem that triggers asthma.

Some people may even be allergic to simple, over-the-counter drugs like aspirin. Once you're sensitized to a substance, later encounters with it will likely stimulate your body to produce chemicals that irritate already-sensitive airways and trigger an attack. But in people with asthma it's difficult to identify the specific allergen. If you suspect that your asthma symptoms may be triggered by allergies, an option is to get tested by an allergy specialist. Knowing what you are allergic to will allow you to practice preventive medicine by avoiding contact as best you can.

## Environment

An important element in triggering asthma attacks is environment. Polluted environments and cold, windy weather exacerbate asthma reactions. Although asthma can occur in any climate, asthmatics who are unusually susceptible to respiratory infections often do better living in warm, temperate areas. Some people even go so far as to move to another part of the country in order to find a drier, warmer, less pollinated or polluted environment. But while seeking the perfect place, asthmatics need to avoid living near golf courses or other areas where the spraying of insecticides can trigger asthmatic symptoms.

## Work Environment

Your work environment also plays a part. A persistent cough and trouble breathing at work suggest job-related, or occupational, asthma, particularly when symptoms worsen toward the end of the day. Irritants in the work environment can include dust, molds, cleaning products, work-related chemicals such as those used for copy machines, and new carpeting and furnishings, which often release formaldehyde, a common asthma trigger. Also, if you work in an office where the air is processed or air conditioned, make sure that the filters are changed regularly.

## Physical Activity

Physical exercise is not only possible but important to the well-being of all asthmatics, yet there are times when strenuous exercise may lead to wheezing and coughing. Called exercise-induced asthma, this reaction affects about one person out of eight and is on the rise. Exercise-induced asthma usually kicks in from five to ten minutes after beginning a steady, hard workout. It's worsened by cold, dry air, which depletes the bronchial tubes of needed warmth and moisture. This cooling and drying out of airways also correlates with the rate of breathing during physical exertion. Besides running, other activities that commonly trigger this syndrome are outdoor cycling and skiing. Preventive measures for exercise-induced asthma will be discussed in chapter 11, along with advice on nutrition and dealing with the environment.

## Respiratory Infection

Medical doctors see respiratory infection as a major trigger. A common cold, bronchitis, flu, or sinus infection can turn difficult and complex when it aggravates airways that are already sensitive. Paying attention to basics, like getting enough rest, eating well, exercising, avoiding allergens and pollutants, and attending to the stress in your life before it becomes overwhelming, is just good common sense and makes for the most effective preventive health care.

## Emotional Stress

The emotional and social aspects of asthmatics' lives are often the most neglected of all irritants. Conventional medicine argues that this disease is not of mental, emotional, or psychological origin; it insists that emotional stress will not trigger asthma attacks unless a person is *already predisposed* to the disease. In fact, the emotional environment is usually overlooked or ignored. It's rare that asthmatics are asked by their doctors to describe what's going on in their lives that might have precipitated an attack. Such things are side issues at best.

For instance, after going through an entire first visit with a pulmonary specialist, Jeff, a thirty-year-old asthmatic, was dismayed that he had not been asked anything about his emotional, social, or spiritual well-being. Physical symptoms and environmental trouble spots had been discussed, but his mental and emotional condition was treated as if nonexistent. When Dr. Renata Engler, chief of the department of allergy and immunology at Walter Reed Medical Center, compiled extensive data on "alternative systems of medical practice," one of her conclusions was that "patients turn to alternative care because they do not feel their physicians listen to their problems."[2] For the most part, conventional medicine ignores the big picture—the one that acknowledges the relevance of the inner life of emotion and spirit as crucial to our health and well-being.

As mentioned earlier, Gerald Epstein, M.D., assistant clinical professor of psychiatry at Mount Sinai Medical Center in New York, has pioneered a very different approach to asthma, one that looks at this disease as a *meaningful phenomenon*. He views the emotional issues in patients' lives as key factors in the illness and is interested in what meaning their lungs have for them. Finding out what was going on at the onset of the asthma can be particularly important in defining this meaning. According to Dr. Epstein, the asthma may be a cry for freedom, or it may be about abandonment or an experience of loss or dependency.[3]

The idea that emotions are intimately tied to health is not a new one. Even before the time of Hippocrates (500 B.C.E.) and up until three hundred years ago when Descartes, the French philosopher, informed the world that the mind and body were separate, physicians believed our emotions played an important role in the genesis of a disease. Yet it's only with the recent research in the area of psychoneuroimmunology (the study of the effects of the mind on the nervous, hormonal, and immune systems) that this connection between mental and physical functions has once again emerged in mainstream medicine. This renewed understanding can be crucial especially in our approach to asthma.

## CONVENTIONAL MEDICINE

Conventional medicine is what most of us grew up with. It has a sense of stability, of authority, of solidity, and of science. All in all, we tend to believe it knows what it's doing. Conventional medicine may be defined, most simply, as medical interventions taught extensively at medical schools in the United States and provided at the hospitals here, while nonconventional medicine is considered to be medical interventions not extensively taught at U.S. medical schools or generally provided at U.S. hospitals. More than anything else, what seems to make a therapy conventional is whether it has been *introduced* by mainstream Western physicians and scientists rather than by "outsiders," particularly those who take their case directly to the public.[4]

Conventional medicine is also known as mainstream, orthodox, regular, scientific, allopathic, Western, or modern medicine. Nonconventional medicine is often called complementary, alternative, unorthodox, irregular, unscientific, and naturopathic. Some of these terms are obviously inappropriate and inflammatory (such as *irregular* and *unscientific*), while others (such as *complementary* and *alternative*) tend to trivialize medicine that is not part of the orthodoxy of the mainstream system.

Surprisingly, the term *allopathy*, which has become a byword of Western medicine over the past thirty years, did not originate in the conventional medical community. In fact, it was coined by a homeopath, Dr. Samuel Hahnemann, who lived between 1755 and 1843.

Hahnemann invented the word *allopathic* to describe the harsh and abusive therapies many of his colleagues used to cause effects different from those of the disease itself. The implication of this term is best understood in the context of the time. In 1790, Hahnemann was disenchanted with the heroic therapies of regular physicians, which included such treatments as emetics, bloodletting, and purging. He viewed these therapies as an outgrowth of the doctrine of contraries, a centuries-old concept that any illness or deviation of normal bodily function could be corrected by applying a counteracting procedure or force.[5]

It's clear that Hahnemann did not mean the term *allopathy* as a compliment, making it particularly ironic that in the lexicon of conventional medicine, this term denotes scientific exclusivity and is held in high regard. Homeopaths, like Hahnemann, approached healing very differently. They treated "like with like," using minute doses of a drug that in massive amounts would produce symptoms in healthy individuals similar to the disease itself. This subtle method brings the system into balance, allowing it to come to terms with its own physiological process by alleviating symptoms in a gentle, nontoxic way.

Of course we are interested in getting rid of the pain and suffering produced by a disease. Yet it's important to know that allopathy, which seeks to suppress or eliminate symptoms and to get rid of the disease as quickly as possible, is neither the only way nor necessarily the best way to do this. Its technological procedures, such as surgery, invasive tests, and strong medications, are aggressive, and the side effects of these may be as devastating to the patient's health as the disease itself. However, this is the kind of treatment on which most people, including asthmatics, depend. Following are categories and types of current allopathic options. These are not meant as recommendations but as information about some of the possibilities available. For a full explanation on how to use the following types of medications and which ones are right for you, consult with your physician.

*Conventional/Allopathic Medications*
- Bronchodilators
- Anti-inflammatories
- Leukotriene modifiers
- Beta-agonists and xanthines
- Anticholergenics
- Antiallergics

Medications are chosen by physicians according to the patient's symptoms, medical history, the physician's clinical experience, and the recommendations of the new national guidelines. In addition to relieving and preventing symptoms, all medications may produce what physicians and pharmacists call side effects. Please note, however, that *side effects* is a misleading term. It makes what may be damaging seem unimportant, prompting you to believe that despite the dangers or discomforts that are present, the benefits of the particular drug take precedence. Before using any of these treatments, make sure that you question your physician thoroughly regarding *all* the possible effects that a drug may have. If you do not receive enough information from your doctor to satisfy you, ask your pharmacist, go to the library, or get on the Internet and do your homework. If there is an emergency situation for which you must be treated immediately, take these steps as soon as possible after the crisis has passed.

## TRADITIONAL AND NATURAL APPROACHES TO ASTHMA

Words are powerful. The way we label things deeply influences our consciousness, thought, and behavior. Therefore, in the rest of the book, *traditional* and *natural* medicine will be used in place of the terms *alternative*, *complementary*, and *nonconventional*, while mainstream Western medicine will be called *conventional* or *allopathic*.

It's important to make this distinction, since the terms *nonconventional, alternative,* and *complementary* are misleading, bound up in the politics of medicine, government, and the insurance and pharmaceutical industries. Although conventional, mainstream medicine is ordinarily referred to as *traditional medicine,* it is still in its infancy compared to systems like homeopathy, Chinese, Ayurvedic, and imagery. *Tradition,* as defined by the *American Heritage Dictionary,* refers to "a mode of thought or behavior followed by a people from generation to generation." Allopathy is less than three hundred years old, and despite its popularity in Westernized countries, it has no long-standing lineage.

"We could learn from the Navajo," says James Dalen, M.D., the editor of *Archives of Internal Medicine.* "The Navajo have integrated *unconventional* Western medicine, which is provided by the Indian Health Service, into their centuries-old *conventional* health care, which is provided by native healers."[6]

It is your perception, perspective, and value system that determine what is true for you. For the Navajo, the truth is rooted in their long history of Native American medicine. For them, this healing tradition is neither alternative nor unconventional. Instead, it is Western medicine that is new and has yet to prove itself.

The genuine traditional systems have a constancy that endures through centuries. Yet, even the most highly praised scientific techniques, medications, or technologies may become obsolete in a relatively short time as new discoveries appear on the scene or as severely damaging effects surface. Think of Thalidomide. This sedative drug was withdrawn from the market but not until after it was found to cause severe birth defects in the fetuses of pregnant women. As for steroids, the "magic bullet" frequently prescribed for asthma, their power to diminish symptoms by reducing inflammation and allergic reaction also brings some dangerous and debilitating effects like severe immune deficiency, low blood sugar, cataracts, osteoporosis, arthritis, high blood pressure, and weight gain.

If you are someone who isn't getting the relief you want, who doesn't like taking drugs, or is concerned about short- or long-term effects, you may want to consider using natural and traditional therapies instead. Interest in natural medicine has been increasing since the 1960s. Currently, since patients are demanding more natural therapies, they are quickly becoming a major influence in the mainstream population.

In 1990, the total expenditure for natural and traditional therapies was 13.7 billion dollars, 10.3 billion of which was paid out of pocket. In the vast majority of cases (89 percent), these visits were not prescribed by a conventional physician, and 72 percent of the patients did not discuss these visits with their doctors.[7] In 1997, Americans made 629 million visits to natural medicine practitioners, more than the number of visits to all primary care physicians.[8]

It's clear that there is a tremendous gap between the kind of treatment people want and what conventional medicine has made available. Recently, some conventional physicians have begun tuning into this disconnection and are asking for scientifically sound data on natural treatments and products.[9] A few are even beginning to recommend drugless therapies to treat chronic illnesses such as asthma. Many natural modalities are ancient in origin and can enhance conventional treatment or even wean some people off drugs completely. Some natural therapies, techniques, and practices that you may want to explore are listed below, while mental imagery, the mindbody treatment of choice that this book prescribes, is introduced here more fully.

*Natural and Traditional Therapies*
- Chinese medicine
- Homeopathy
- Ayurvedic medicine
- Reflexology
- Yoga
- Massage

## MENTAL IMAGERY

Mental imagery, sometimes called visualization, is the language used by the mind to communicate with the body. This ancient, self-empowering, healing technique can be used on your own or with the supervision of an experienced guide. Unlike hypnosis, which puts you in a deeply relaxed state that causes you to be open to the suggestions of others, imagery enlivens you. When you engage in imagery, you feel relaxed on the outside yet more alert and awake on the inside. Thus it gives you a sense of greater control and awareness.

When you close your eyes, do a simple breathing process, and turn your attention inward, you feel an immediate shift. Even the simplest image (such as seeing yourself inhaling clear blue light through your nose and releasing dark gray smoke through your mouth), can be employed as a tool for relaxation and relieving symptoms. Once you begin to delve more deeply into this practice, you can then move beyond symptom relief toward healing the core issues involved in asthma as well as in other illnesses and challenging life situations.

One of the many extraordinary benefits of imagery is its ability to create healing changes in a very short time. Just a minute or two of imagery can have a positive effect. Another advantage is the ease with which one can use it. This simple practice can be engaged in anywhere, anytime, and without much preparation. Often, people who just begin using imagery get immediate results. When you feel an asthma symptom coming on, imagery can be used as a deterrent; in the case of a full-blown attack it can be a powerful ally for calming you and for abating the attack.

In even the most challenging circumstances, imagery continually demonstrates its power—a power that creates no ill side effects. Later, in chapter 4, you will learn exactly how to incorporate this healing technique into your own life on a daily basis. Now, in the following chapter, you can make the impossible possible, as you begin to redefine asthma and transform the asthma monster into a friend.

# CHAPTER 3

# REDEFINING YOUR RELATIONSHIP WITH ASTHMA

*Man is made by his beliefs. As he believes so he is.*
BHAGAVAD GITA

Redefining your relationship with asthma may seem like a monumental task. But with the help of this hands-on approach, it becomes not only possible, but FUN. By way of a simple awareness technique, we demonstrate how to prevent panic at the first signs of an attack. You then learn to redirect your thinking so as to redefine and transform the place that asthma has assumed in your life. In addition, the mindbody questionnaire that you will find at the end of the chapter asks two pivotal questions that can change your entire outlook. If you do nothing else but read this section and integrate what it proposes, you will already be well on your way to living an asthma-free life.

The following story invites you to accompany Nora, a participant in the FUN program, through a private session with Kathy, then through an asthma attack and beyond.

Nora is a forty-year-old woman who has been at war with asthma for most of her life. Not long ago she went through a bitter divorce that sapped most of her resources. She also made a career change that left her feeling disappointed and unfulfilled. Now once again this disease has gained the upper hand.

"Sometimes a year or two goes by and my asthma is fine," Nora told Kathy during her first session. "But then something stressful happens, and out of the blue it's back. Even the medications can't seem to control it. And I always wind up feeling even more stressed out, frustrated, and disappointed. Like I've failed."

## ANATOMY OF NORA'S ASTHMA ATTACK

At the earliest sign of what even *might* be an asthma symptom, Nora begins to feel she has no control over what's going on and that she's in life-threatening danger. This feeling is born of her long-held belief that asthma is synonymous with suffocation and death. Out of habit she succumbs to these anxious thoughts, and her body's response is to send a barrage of nerve impulses to the cells that line her airways. Since Nora is predisposed to hyperactivity in these airways, these impulses easily trigger the bronchial constriction that precipitates a sense of tightness in her chest and difficulty breathing. As the vicious cycle continues, her tension further constricts the flow of air going in and out and produces symptoms that become progressively worse.

Nora's distress, provoked by her belief that her life is in danger and that she "could die," produces a cascade of biological events. These events exacerbate the symptom, real or not, and soon escalate into a genuine attack. Essentially, Nora's body goes into a state of emergency, and what begins as a mild symptom soon spirals into a full-blown asthma attack. The muscles lining the airways tighten; the lining of the bronchial tubes swells and becomes inflamed; and the mucus that lubricates the airways becomes thick and sticky, sometimes plugging them up. It gets more and more difficult to exhale, with air depleted of oxygen having become trapped in the lungs, leaving no room for fresh air to enter.[1]

Nora's response is best explained by the new field of cognitive neuropsychology called "expectancy theory." Quite simply, this branch of psychology makes a scientific case for our beliefs and expectations having a significant impact on our physical reality. Interestingly, it parallels the ancient, mystical principle, often ridiculed by the scientific community, that says our thoughts and beliefs create our reality. Expectancy theory contends that our conditioned responses occur almost instantly with no apparent conscious thought and are hardwired into the brain. Since our lives are filled with ambiguity, what's *perceived* as dangerous produces the same results as what actually *is* dangerous.[2] Quite simply, what the brain *believes* about the immediate future is perceived as true! Thus, what may be only a mild asthma symptom, or even what is perceived to be a symptom, becomes a lifethreatening event, first in the person's mind, then in actuality.

However, no matter how serious or debilitating your illness, once you understand that this connection of body and mind exists, there is always hope. Dr. Betty Wray, the former president of the American College of Allergy, Asthma, and Immunology, has stated that while medication can be a crucial element of any treatment plan, it's often not enough. She agrees that asthma is a mental issue as well as a physical one and believes that what you think, feel, and affects your actual experience of the disease.[3]

When Kathy asked Nora if she was willing to explore a new way to deal with the asthma—a way that required paying attention to what her symptom was trying to tell her instead of sending her body frightening messages about an outcome she couldn't really predict—Nora readily agreed. At this point Kathy shared two important things with her that could short-circuit her habitual panic pattern and change her relationship to this disease forever.

- The first was to stop calling it "my" asthma and instead to call it "the" asthma.
- The second was to stop viewing asthma and its symptoms as the "enemy" and to begin seeing it as a "friend."

Nora looked at Kathy as if she were out of her mind. "I can't do it," she said. "How can I treat it as a friend when I feel like it's some monster out to destroy me?" Kathy reminded Nora that mindbody medicine doesn't view symptoms as random or meaningless—it's not the *asthma monster* but the *belief monster* that holds her hostage. When as asthmatics we see this disease as the enemy, we set up an adversarial relationship, both with the asthma and with ourselves. This prevents us from hearing the message the symptoms are trying to convey. But when we stop labeling it "monster" and telling it to "shut up," we give the body and the asthma the opportunity to express themselves and to impart their healing message.

Kathy then advised Nora that this work is optional. She is free to do it or not. Making this choice is part of becoming her own authority, a crucial factor in the mindbody approach. The next time she has an attack or senses one coming on, she can use this new way of thinking as a tool for panic prevention. The instructions for doing this are simple:

---

## SSTUFF:
## EXERCISE FOR PANIC PREVENTION

*Intention:* To prevent and short-circuit the panic response experienced at the onset of asthma symptoms.

*Frequency:* Every time you notice what feels like a symptom coming on.

At the moment of noticing a symptom, simply take out your notebook or journal (one we advise that you keep just for this work), and in writing describe your SSTUFF. SSTUFF stands for:

The **S**ituation you are in (where you are, what's going on, who you're with).

---

The **S**ensations you are feeling in your body.

The **T**houghts you are thinking now and the Thoughts you were thinking before the symptom began.

The **U** represents YOU. It's here to remind you that U are not the symptom. Because you are not the symptom, you can stop, step aside, watch, and take charge instead of being swept away by panic.

The **F**eelings you are feeling now.

The **F**eelings you were feeling before the symptom began.

Prepare your notebook beforehand by writing down the categories for SSTUFF and leaving spaces after them so you are ready.

Situation:

_____

Sensations:

_____

Thoughts:

_____

Feelings:

_____

If you take time out to deal with your SSTUFF whenever breathing difficulties start, you will soon be able to identify recurring personal patterns that relate to the onset of symptoms. This alone often is enough to begin making a difference. In *Space, Time and Medicine*, Larry Dossey, M.D., a forerunner in the field of mindbody work, cites a study in which chronic headache sufferers were asked to keep a diary of the frequency and severity of their headaches. Inexplicably, when they began to keep the diary the headaches disappeared.[4]

One morning not long after this session, Nora awoke at 2:00 A.M. with a tight feeling in her chest. The inhaler was nearby on her dresser, but as she was about to reach for it she hesitated, remembering she had a choice. At that instant she reversed her tendency and picked up her notebook instead. She opened it and started writing about her SSTUFF. She described the Situation: *waking up alone in her bedroom in the middle of the night.* The Sensations: *constriction in her chest and the heaviness and constriction in her daily life.* Her Thoughts: *fear of the asthma symptom and of needing the medication to survive.* Her Thoughts of the future: *that this will always interfere with her life.* Her Feelings: *anger about the limitations this illness imposes* and her Feelings of *frustration concerning the stultifying relationship* she has been in for the past three years.

As Nora wrote about her sensations, thoughts, and feelings, a transformation began. The tightness in her chest started to lessen, her breathing became easier, and the walls of her room no longer seemed as if they were closing in on her. Instead there was a sense of space in which she could actually move and breathe. At this point, Nora had arrived at a place where she and the asthma had the opportunity to form a different relationship, one that could go beyond anxiety, fear, and frustration and finally allow her to make some sense out of what was going on.

What's going on now with *you* as you read this? If you find yourself feeling tense or resistant, thinking, "That's fine for *her*, but it couldn't possibly work for me," stop for a moment and ask yourself: How am I doing so far with this illness? Chances are, the "asthma monster" is still a threat in (and to) your life. Of course, taking a new approach that involves breaking your habitual response to your symptoms will seem foreign and uncomfortable. But redefining your relationship with asthma is a matter of *life and breath.* Since each of us has a special relationship with this disease, we have included a questionnaire at the end of this chapter to help you discover what that relationship is.

By using this questionnaire you will be taking an important

step toward:

- Creating a responsible relationship with asthma
- Paying attention to the asthma and the way you respond to it
- Making a transition from illness to health

Wherever you are right now with this disease is the perfect place to start. A shift in your stance (including your beliefs, attitudes, feelings, thoughts, and behaviors), no matter how small, will act as a catalyst for change. Focusing on the asthma in this new way will enable you to create your own self-care program, one based on a personalized, compassionate kind of medicine that's not easy to come by in the conventional system. What's more, by changing your relationship with yourself and the asthma, you are bound to gain valuable understanding regarding all areas of your life.

## PREPARING TO USE THE ASTHMA QUESTIONNAIRE

Instead of offering you a conventional questionnaire that explores cause-and-effect relationships, we have chosen to show you how asking simple questions can quickly reveal profound truths. Though in our ordinary state of awareness life appears static, with every incident, circumstance, and person entirely separate from every other, in fact, it is not. Life flows together in one continuous movement of which asthma is a part. Thus it makes no sense to look at the asthma as a separate entity. The following questions will help you to see this illness within the context of your whole life. Viewing asthma this way instead of as an alien threat, you can begin to understand its meaning and finally see the previously two-dimensional picture of this disease in three dimensions.

As you answer the questions, if any of them provoke feelings of anxiety, sensations of constriction, or an uncomfortable change in breathing, stop and jot down what you experience. Making note of the questions that bring up these feelings or sensations will enable you to see the intimate relationship of body, breath, and mind. Whatever your response (mental or physical), it's valuable. There is no standard to adhere to, no right or wrong, no normal or abnormal. Be kind to yourself. Allow this questionnaire to act as a healing tool that you refer to whenever you want or need it. And let this be your first step in living life with a greater sense of connection, freedom, and joy.

## THE MINDBODY ASTHMA QUESTIONNAIRE

### Section I
1. When were you first diagnosed with asthma?
2. What was happening in your life and in the life of your family around this time?
3. What most concerns you about the asthma and its symptoms?
4. How do you respond to attacks and symptoms?
5. Who else is involved in your care? In what way? How do you feel about this?

### Section II
When an asthma attack (or symptom) occurs:
1. Where are you?
2. Who are you with?
3. What are you doing?
4. What is happening?
5. What are you thinking and feeling?

### Section III
1. How does asthma affect your life?
2. Does the asthma serve any purpose?
3. What are you willing to sacrifice (change, let go of, release) so you can live asthma free—what job, person, belief, habit, place, story, and so forth?

Note: *Though* sacrifice *seems to be a dirty word in our society, for thousands of years it has been considered a healing practice. Sacrifice simply means letting go of something you value in order to obtain something of higher or greater value. Think of a sacrifice hit in baseball. The hitter makes a sacrifice so the runner can score. Makes sense, doesn't it?*

## Section IV

Here you suspend all disbelief for a few moments and imagine living a new life, one without asthma. Answer these questions spontaneously. Let your first thoughts be the ones that guide you. Just relax, and let it flow from your heart. Then write and/or draw your response.

1. In this new life, what are you doing?
2. How does it feel?
3. What is different about you, about your life?

In other words, how do you think it would be for you to enjoy life, completely healed? Allow this to become a mental image for a minute, and implant it in your mind—not as a wish, a thought, or an idea, but as an actual felt, seen, and lived experience of the imagination. Then set this image and questionnaire aside. When you are ready, go on to chapter 4. There you will learn to enjoy the practice of mental imagery, a technique to use even under the most trying circumstances. If you are looking for a way to reduce medication and free yourself from symptoms within a short time period, the next chapter is meant for you. In addition, by learning to use this technique, you can begin to make healing changes in every area of your life.

# CHAPTER 4

# MIND MEDICINE

## Tapping into the Power of Imagination

*Imagination is more important than knowledge, for knowledge is limited while imagination embraces the entire world.*
ALBERT EINSTEIN

At the core of every image is a picture, and every picture is worth a thousand words. The tree, the lake, the sky appear in our minds instantaneously, yet to each of us they may appear different. The tree may be sturdy, willowy, leafless, or lush; the lake may be muddy or crystal clear; the sky may be a brilliant blue, sunset pink, or a darkening gray. What you see imparts a feeling and reveals your beliefs. These feelings and beliefs can be calming or energizing, disturbing or painful. They may encourage or deter you from your present course in life; they may generate ecstasy or sadness, joy or anger. Whatever you see and feel holds value for you, even when it is unsettling. Imagery gives you the opportunity to observe, change, and consciously choose your beliefs, thoughts, and feelings, without discussion or analysis, thereby saving yourself time and a great deal of unnecessary worry while creating immediate benefits. In the following story you will see how Sandra used imagery to deal with asthma symptoms and how her experience went well beyond the benefits offered by conventional medication.

## SOLUTIONS FOR SYMPTOMS THROUGH IMAGERY

Sandra, a forty-three-year-old attorney, has been asthmatic since childhood. Despite using a variety of approaches, she has always felt enslaved to her disease. She has tried both ignoring her condition and catering to it. Yet, though everything seems to help for a time, nothing gives her the release she seeks. She is tired of searching for a solution that constantly evades her. Feeling drained and confused, she decides to use imagery as a treatment of last resort.

Sandra closes her eyes, turns her senses inward, and does some reverse breathing (exhaling first though her mouth, then inhaling through her nose). With this simple preparation, she enters the world of her imagination where anything is possible. Here there are no rules, no diagnoses or prognoses—in fact, no limitations of any kind. Using an imagery exercise called "Liberation from Slavery" (you can find it in chapter 8), Sandra sees and feels herself chained to her illness, which appears to her as a large beast pressing her down, its foot planted firmly on her chest. Uncomfortable as this image may be, once she sees it she has the opportunity to acknowledge it (in effect, to *turn toward it*) and to make a change. Using her imagination, she finds a key that unlocks the chains, breaks free of the beast, and releases herself from its power. Suddenly the beast begins shrinking while Sandra grows taller. As the chains fall away, the restriction and heaviness in her chest diminish. She feels lighter, her breathing becomes easier, and the sense of fear and powerlessness she had been feeling is replaced by hope and clarity.

The benefits Sandra derived from doing this exercise were far-reaching and immediate. Her imagery was a mirror that revealed her from the inside out. Instantly, she learned truths about herself that until now she had overlooked, even denied. Indeed, she was stronger, "taller," and more powerful than she ever suspected. By freeing herself from the chains (her beliefs and fears about the power the illness had over her life), she became bigger than this disease, something she had always felt was too much for her to handle.

By using the key to release herself, she affected her beliefs, thoughts, and feelings in a positive and liberating way. Thus she went far beyond ordinary thinking, where such things are "impossible," and became her own authority, the one who is ultimately in control of her choices.

Sandra's experience is not uncommon. With a little practice, you too can learn to do this for yourself. The warm-up exercises below give you a simple way to begin. Before doing them, however, take time to look over the next section. Here you will find the information that can easily help you to get started with the process.

## PREPARING TO IMAGE

Preparing to image involves turning from the outer, material world toward the inner, invisible one—from everyday life to the life within, where your deepest knowledge and your natural healing powers are waiting for you to find them. Preparation involves paying attention to the following items:

- Timing
- Position
- Intention
- Breathing and relaxation
- Attitude

### Timing
The three best times to do imagery are: in the morning right after getting out of bed (after urinating, before having breakfast), at twilight, and at the end of the day before going to sleep. When you begin in the morning, you set the tone for the day. By doing it in the evening you complete the day. With most exercises you will continue for 21 days, then take seven days off, and if necessary do another cycle for another 21 days.

## Position

Find a quiet place where you can relax without interruption. Sit in a comfortable chair with armrests (if possible). Keep your feet and legs uncrossed, flat on the floor, your arms on the armrests or relaxed on your thighs, and your back and head erect. This is called the pharaoh's position, since it was used by Egyptian royalty to contact inner guides. We don't advise lying down to do imagery unless you are injured or ill. Too often, people become groggy and fall asleep. In most instances, unless you are working to relieve insomnia, the intention of imagery is to wake yourself up, to become alert, alive, rejuvenated, reborn.

## Intention

Close your eyes and state your intention to yourself. This means that you silently tell yourself what it is that you want. Your intention should be clear, brief, and to the point. For example, your intention might be to breathe freely, to heal asthma, to become more relaxed, to reduce medication, to develop more confidence, or even to run a marathon.

## Breathing and Relaxation

The brief breathing preparation included here helps you to become quiet and relaxed yet stay awake and aware. It may even be used on its own as a mini–relaxation process. First, with eyes closed, you begin to pay attention to your breath, just as it is. Then you consciously begin to breathe rhythmically and easily, in through your nose and out through your mouth, allowing your exhalations gradually to become longer and slower than your inhalations. Now you exhale one long, easy breath through your mouth (no need to force it), then inhale a shorter breath through your nose. Do this "out-in" breathing (first *out* through the mouth, then *in* through your nose) two more times.

Starting with the *exhalation* may be unfamiliar, but it calms and centers you. It helps draw your attention away from the outside life and directs you toward the life within. Once you have completed this process, return to your normal breathing and do the imagery exercise. At the end of the exercise, you breathe out one more time and then open your eyes.

Note: *Breathing out longer than breathing in stimulates the vagus nerve, the major quieting nerve in the body, which originates in the medulla, at the base of the brain. This nerve branches to the heart, lungs, and intestinal tract, slowing the heart rate and pulse, lowering blood pressure, and calming muscular contractions of the intestines.*[1]

## Breathing Recap

At the beginning of almost every imagery exercise, you will see the words *Breathe out three times.* This does not mean that you exhale one time after the other, without breathing in. Instead, it's a brief way of saying what we just explained above.

1. Breathe out a single long exhalation through your mouth.
2. Breathe in through your nose.
3. Do this two more times (out through the mouth, in through the nose).
4. Return to normal breathing and proceed with the imagery.
5. Breathe out at the end of the exercise and open your eyes.

## Attitude

Imagery work involves commitment to the process and the discipline to remain in the present moment. There's no need to concern yourself about results; you do it and let it go. Becoming concerned with the outcome—worrying about whether it will work, how soon, how well, and so forth—is a self-defeating habit used in trying to control things and "figure them out." It steals you away from the present and pushes you into the future. Since the imagination is limitless and anything is possible, your logical mind cannot analyze what's going on in your imagery. Save your energy for more productive things. Should your mind drift during the imagery, refocus your attention by breathing out again, one time, through your mouth.

Remember to stay open and nonjudgmental. Your imagery is unique, it's yours alone. It's neither good nor bad, normal nor abnormal. Some exercises may slightly shock you or make you feel uncomfortable, while others infuse you with a sense of joy, freedom, and lightness. Although you may not believe it now, the discomfort or shock is not "bad"; it's just as valuable as the joy. Without it, we would not be able to recognize what we must do in order to heal.

## WARM-UPS: A BRIEF INTRODUCTION TO IMAGERY

The simple exercises that follow are short warm-ups that are easy to do. You might think of them as calisthenics of the mind; they are a pleasant introduction to the healing exercises we will share with you later in this chapter and throughout the book. These exercises involve all the senses: seeing, hearing, smelling, tasting, and touching. This is why we call the process *imagery* instead of visualization, which refers only to the sense of sight. You may want someone to read these to you; or you can put them on tape (as you can do with any imagery exercise). Another option is to do one exercise at a time, opening your eyes after each to read the one that comes next. This gives you some practice in traveling quickly, back and forth, in and out of your imagination.

*To Begin*
1. Find a comfortable, seated position, in a quiet space.
2. Close your eyes and turn your attention inward.
3. Focus gently and rhythmically on your breathing, as directed above.
4. Once you complete this process, which takes no more than a minute or so, return to your normal breathing and begin to image.

Now imagine the following, spending only a few seconds on each:

1. See before you a familiar face.
2. See a friendly animal coming toward you.
3. See yourself walking along a mountain path.
4. See a calm lake reflecting the starry sky above.
5. Hear rain beating down on the roof and against the windows.
6. Hear a dog barking.
7. Hear children laughing and playing.
8. Smell the saltwater air at the beach.
9. Smell the scent of a rose or your favorite flower.
10. Imagine cutting open a lemon and sucking on it.
11. Taste the sticky, smooth sweetness of a spoonful of honey.
12. Imagine turning on the water faucet, filling a glass with cool water, and drinking it.
13. Feel a piece of satin against your face.
14. Feel the sand of an ocean beach beneath your feet and between your toes.
15. Open a package of balloons and choose one of any color. Blow up the balloon, tie it with a golden string, let it rise above your head, and don't let go. See what happens.

Once you have finished, take a few moments to notice which senses are strongest for you and which need some practice. If you find it difficult to see things in your imagination, begin looking more closely at things in your daily life; observe them in detail and with a deeper appreciation. If you are unable to hear, start listening in a more active way. If you do not enjoy a keen sense of smell or taste or touch, begin honing these senses in your daily experience. You might wish to record these impressions in your notebook. You will find that as you go on with the work, your ability to image will improve.

# IMAGERY: A PERSONAL RESOURCE FOR POWER

According to *The Barrett Power Theory*, developed by Elizabeth Barrett, coordinator at the Center for Nursing Research at Hunter College in New York, power is the "freedom to make *aware choices* regarding life situations, including health-promoting changes"[2] (emphasis added). By consciously choosing to use imagery as a tool for creating change, Sandra and now you have tapped into the four inter-related dimensions described by Barrett in her work: awareness, choice, the freedom to act intentionally, and involvement in creating change. This revitalizing experience served Sandra well. It enabled her to deal effectively, not only with the asthma, but with all obstacles in her path, for it assured her that she could reverse the power struc-ture between herself and the asthma beast. Using imagery disarmed her fear, fortified her will, and moved her to take action. In approach-ing her difficulty by using imagery instead of only conventional med-ications, whose long-term effects concerned and debilitated her, Sandra began to generate a new belief system, one that provides infi-nite possibilities. And all this happened *in less than three minutes*.

Since the technique of imagery can quickly help you to gener-ate a sense of personal power and strength, we have chosen to introduce it early on. Like Sandra, we are all imprisoned by our beliefs, which, though invisible to us, are as strong and limiting as the bars of a cell. For one person such a belief might be as simple and deadly as "This disease will probably kill me." For another it might be a self-judgment that insists "I don't deserve to be loved." For someone else it might be "I need her, his, or their approval to feel I'm okay."

Both a potent mind technology and the mental equivalent of a laser, imagery cuts quickly, deeply, and precisely through the layers of mental armor that prevent us from living authentically, vividly revealing our beliefs and emotions without analysis or discussion. For many of our clients it has been the golden key that opens the door to freedom. Exploring the world of imagination is an exciting, valuable, and life-transforming journey; one that enables you to truly see yourself, perhaps for the first time. Once this happens, all levels of your existence have the potential to be reborn, renewed, and healed.

Although you will learn many valuable techniques in this book, imagery lies at the heart of this program, giving you access to this imaginal world where anything is possible. Engaging the mind, body, and spirit, imagery serves as a catalyst for turning the lead of illness into the gold of healing. Using this process makes what seems impossible, beyond what you ordinarily can accomplish, into a challenge that invigorates and strengthens you from the inside out. This brings life into focus in a new and harmonious way.

## RESEARCH STUDY WITH ASTHMATICS
## DEMONSTRATES POWERFUL RESULTS

The importance and potency of imagery as a technique for alleviating asthma was demonstrated in a research study funded by the Office of Alternative Medicine of the National Institutes of Health at Lenox Hill Hospital in New York City. The study compared an asthma control group using no imagery with the asthma patients who did use imagery. It demonstrated that 47 percent of the asthmatics in the imagery group significantly decreased or discontinued medication *without compromising pulmonary function*. None reported side effects; these statistics signaled that the imagery had a substantial positive result. The corresponding figure for the control group, however, was just 18 percent, and here patients were able only to decrease, not discontinue, medication. Patients also reported that using the imagery technique led them to new insights and feelings regarding the possibility of freedom, happiness, and health. Through the practice of imagery they realized that the mind is powerful and can change all aspects of life, not just asthma.[3] The following statements by participants in the study express these feelings clearly:

"I was able to direct my attention inward . . . and tap into inner resources, talents, and strengths that were dormant and unused due to fear, anxiety, and low self-esteem."

"I experienced a personal crisis. . . . Imagery relieved my stress and centered me. Somehow the crisis lessened and I was left with a sense of hope."

"Imagery has given me a tool . . . the ability to participate in my own therapy from within—it has opened new doors and aware-nesses."

Overall, when used consistently by the participants in this study, imagery promoted feelings of safety, security, and powerfulness.

## AN ANCIENT FORM OF MEDICINE RETURNS TO FAVOR

The practice of imagery is simple and direct. It offers you a form of mind medicine that affects the body-mind and creates a bridge to spirit. In many cultures, the imagination has been a primary healing tool for hundreds, even thousands, of years. Beginning in ancient Egypt, it was the medical treatment of choice. Preverbal and univer-sal, imagery was the first language; therefore, it was the first mode of communication, as evidenced by the hieroglyphs on the Egyptian pyramids where pictorial symbols were used to represent meanings or sounds. Considered essential for healing both physical and mental problems, imagery continued to be widely practiced until the mid–seventeenth century by physicians with their patients and by many who chose to use it as a personal therapy. It was then that Descartes's dualistic theory of the mind as separate from the body gained dominion in Western thought. From this point on mind med-icine, of which imagery had always been a part, fell into disrepute. Yet, even during these past three hundred years, while allopathic medicine and physical science have gained tremendous favor and dominance, mental imagery (or what is sometimes called visualiza-tion) was still used by many who never forgot its power.

Recently, things have taken a promising turn: imagery and mindbody medicine in general have resurfaced and increased in popularity. Mainstream medicine has begun to notice that the mind and our emotional states may indeed alter and even determine the course of a physical illness—that treating emotional distress can improve physical health. The imagery study with asthmatics we described earlier is convincing proof of this.

Currently, imagery techniques are being used in some of the most highly respected medical institutions throughout the country to assist in the healing of a wide range of physical ailments including cancer, heart disease, asthma, arthritis, and chronic pain. What for centuries had been thought impossible by conventional sources—the mind generating positive physiological changes in the body—is finally proving a reality, as demonstrated in the story you are about to read.

## Gail and the Golden Inhaler

Gail first tried imagery when she was using both Ventolin and Theophylline; she had been asthmatic for eighteen years. During her most recent attack, which she had a week after her wedding, she had been admitted to the emergency room. A month later, when she saw a sign at the neighborhood YWCA asking for asthmatics to join the research study we just described, Gail jumped right in. She wanted to get off her medications, and using imagery sounded promising. Within a few weeks from the time she began doing the "Golden Inhaler," one of the exercises that was part of the study protocol, Gail told her doctor she was ready to stop the Theophylline and reduce the Ventolin. When he said no to both, she never went back to him again. Gail did, however, get full pulmonary workups throughout the research study, every third week. But she never used Theophylline again and uses Ventolin only rarely.

The following exercise is the one Gail used that helped her turn the corner and release herself from the steady use of medication and her attachment to her inhaler:

# THE GOLDEN INHALER [4] ✳

*Intention:* To give you a way to reduce or replace the use of your regular inhaler.

*Frequency:* Use this exercise as needed or whenever you reach for your regular inhaler. It gives you a choice and helps you to become your own authority.

*Note: There is no introductory breathing process for this exercise.*

Whenever you need to use the inhaler, reach for it, hold it in your hand, and then stop for an instant. In that instant of stopping (and before you do anything with the inhaler), close your eyes and imagine that you are bringing a golden inhaler into your mouth, or however you use it. Take the number of puffs that you ordinarily use, and see this coming out as a blue spray, which you ingest. See it filling your lungs and bronchi with blue light, allowing you to breathe normally. Then open your eyes and complete the action in any way you see fit. (Use the inhaler or don't use the inhaler.)

Gail said that the imagery did more than remove the physical symptom; it allowed her to see connections between her asthma attacks, especially the more severe ones, and her life circumstances. "It's always about transitions—separating from someone or something and going on to another phase in my life," she said. Gail also felt that the imagery had facilitated a change with her mother, "who doesn't like independence in family members, especially in me." Gail feels more separate now. "When we talk I say what I'm feeling, and I let her be herself, without getting upset by her judgments and advice." For Gail, this experience was about becoming her own authority regarding both her medical treatment and her relationship with her mom.

Although Gail quickly dispensed with all medication, in particular her inhaler, all of us need to do this at our own pace, without pressuring ourselves with "stories" about success or failure. As with any of the exercises, state your intention, do it, and see what happens. Even without making the radical change that Gail did, having this exercise at your disposal can provide you with a valuable sense of control and empowerment.

## EVEN THE MOST SERIOUSLY ILL BENEFIT FROM IMAGERY

In a research study done through the Department of Complementary Medicine at Columbia Presbyterian Medical Center in New York, it was demonstrated that even the most seriously ill can benefit from imagery.[5] Heart failure patients, waiting for transplants, attended group imagery sessions once a week for three weeks and practiced the imagery at home every day. Patients with this disease find it virtually impossible to live a normal life. Their dependence on medication, their severely limited physical abilities, and their ambivalence over wanting a new heart—fearing the surgery, wishing for the heart to become available, yet knowing that only someone else's death can make that possible—create a very unstable situation, both medically and emotionally.

Initially, most of the participants in this group were skeptical. What possible good could come of closing their eyes and imagining a beneficial change when even the most advanced technology and best medications had already failed? Yet even this brief taste of imagery that included exercises for improving pulmonary function, physical strength, and emotional resilience created an improvement in their quality of life, as revealed by a test administered once the study was done. The patients voiced their enthusiasm for the treatment by asking for a continuing imagery group, and some of their personal reactions included the following:

"On Wednesday, the weather was terrible. I was walking to the corner store and felt discomfort in my chest area. I had become short of breath, so I sat down on the stoop of a building and started to image. By the time I finished, which was only thirty seconds later, I was feeling great."

"I walk up and down stairs more easily now and am able to walk longer distances without pain. Guided imagery changed my thinking, decreased my pain, . . . and increased my energy."

"I played eighteen holes of golf last weekend with some friends. They couldn't believe it. In between each hole I would stop and do the 'Golden Bellows' exercise—seeing my lungs compressing and pushing out gray smoke, then expanding and filling with light. I never felt short of breath, and I played better than I have in years. I'm sure it was the imagery that did it."

Although this study was applied to patients with heart failure, not asthma, it reinforces the value of using imagery to develop a stance of optimism and empowerment instead of depression and powerlessness—even when a condition has been diagnosed as "medically irreversible."

The "Golden Bellows" exercise, mentioned above, is something you can begin to use for yourself right now. It is a way of breathing, both imaginally and physically, which increases lung strength and capacity, and a way of strengthening the diaphragm.

---

### THE GOLDEN BELLOWS[6]✻

*Intention:* To strengthen and heal the respiratory system. To increase lung capacity.

*Frequency:* If you are experiencing respiratory discomfort, use once every hour or two while awake, up to two minutes at a time. If breathing is normal, use once in morning and once at night.

Close your eyes and breathe out three times. Imagine your lungs as a pair of golden bellows. As you breathe in, see, sense, and feel the bellows filling with white light and expanding. See and feel your chest expanding at the same time.

As you exhale, see the bellows contracting forcibly, pushing out the impure air through your mouth. See this air being emitted as gray smoke and drifting away into the atmosphere. At the same time, see and sense your chest contracting. Now repeat this process up to five more times before opening your eyes. As you do this, know that your lungs are working rhythmically, filling you with energy and life. Then open your eyes and return.

## ENGAGING THE LANGUAGE OF THE HEART

As you have already experienced, when using mental imagery you close your eyes, turn your senses inward, and begin to think in pictures instead of words. With these pictures (or images), your thoughts, beliefs, and feelings are mirrored back to you, and the nature of your illness or difficulty takes on a unique visual form. By working with this form via your imagination, you have the opportunity to make any necessary corrections and enact an immediate change.

While the logical mind figures things out one step at a time, imagery engages the intuitive mind, the part of you that knows wholly, immediately—that speaks a unique personal language, the language of the heart. Like the laser beam we previously mentioned, imagery bypasses ordinary thought, cuts through obstacles, and has the ability to mitigate fears and doubts. It illuminates even the most difficult problems, revealing all at once what you need to know instead of picking things apart, dissecting, testing, diagnosing, and evaluating. By choosing to honor this comprehensive knowledge, you are able to turn toward your difficulty and get in touch with the part of yourself that many people call the inner voice, or the healer within.

For those skeptics who think the term *healer within* sounds New Age-y, pretentious, or unrealistic, stop for a moment and remember how your body naturally heals a cut, a bruise, a sore throat, a muscle pull, even a broken toe or rib. Most of us don't run to the doctor every time we experience a physical difficulty. Yet somehow our bodies know what to do and how to do it, even without prescription medication or expert advice. Imagery picks up on this natural body-mind process and helps it along by sending messages that further inspire, inform, and remind this wise and truthful part of yourself to help you in ways it may not yet be doing.

## Hieroglyphs, Holograms, and Imagination

Egypt is a place rich in its imaginal heritage. Hieroglyphic writing is everywhere. These stylized drawings of people and symbols carved into the stones are an ancient language (a language of images, all having multiple meanings). This pictorial writing give a strong sense of imagery's ancient roots. It reminds us that imagery was a highly valued practice in the Egyptian culture and had far-reaching importance as a language that is both nonverbal and universal.

Like hieroglyphs, holograms are familiar to many of us in a limited way. We have seen holographic images imprinted on objects for years. These images seem to move (turning, opening their eyes, smiling, and so forth) and to have more than the two dimensions that ordinary flat surfaces provide. For the most part, we enjoy them as an oddity, an amusement. But there is a lot more to holograms than this, especially as they relate to imagery and health. Simply put, the hologram[7] is a three-dimensional hieroglyph of the mind. Through their imagery holograms and hieroglyphs convey far more than what we see on the surface: they reveal a wealth of hidden information about our personal natures, histories, health, relationships, and direction in life. Thinking in images instead of words involves thinking holographically—our minds expand past logic and linear thought, moving into an all-at-once mode that relays messages and information instantaneously. Thus, even one brief image can be life changing and reveal many facets of who and what we are.

In the next story, we see how Cheryl, a fifty-year-old asthmatic, used her imagination as a starting point for correcting a family hologram that stood in the way of her healing.


## A FAMILY AFFAIR

Cheryl stated her intentions as wanting to get rid of her asthma, to move forward in her life, and to focus more strongly on her spiritual development. In her imagery she saw a weight on her chest, in the form of an anvil, that restricted her breathing. She then saw a band of angels who appeared and easily lifted the anvil, thus releasing her breath and setting her free. She continued to practice this imagery exercise, and in the following days the anvil transformed and became her mother. Then, as can happen only in imagination, along came Cheryl's dead grandmother, who grabbed her mom by the scruff of her neck and carried her off. Cheryl described her mother as "kicking and screaming, stunned that Grandma could do such a thing." Cheryl's mom had always been abusive, particularly toward Grandma, so Cheryl felt Grandma was dishing out just deserts and was still watching over her.

Through the imagery, what emerged were Cheryl's beliefs and feelings about herself, the asthma, and the possibilities of life. The angels revealed her connection to the invisible world and the life of spirit. The second part of her imagery was a powerful hologram of the mother/daughter issues that for generations had needed correcting in Cheryl's family. Cheryl's image of her mother sitting on top of her then being dragged off, kicking and screaming, revealed the whole restricting and volatile family issue she had been living out her entire life. Cheryl's imagery showed in an instant what had been, what is, and what may be in the future. It revealed, all at once, the connection between her restrictive family situation and the restriction of her breathing. However, the powerful upward movement of her imagery lightened that load and showed the potential for freeing herself from the family error.

Why not try this exercise for yourself and see what *you* discover? What does your own weight look like, and how does it feel when you remove it?

---

## TAKING A WEIGHT OFF YOUR CHEST [8]✳

*Intention:* To alleviate and remove symptoms of asthma.

*Frequency:* Every day for 21 days, for no longer than two minutes. Or use anytime you sense constriction or weight on your chest.

Close your eyes and breathe out three times. See and sense a weight on and in your chest.

Feel and sense the constriction this gives you. Breathe out one time slowly and remove this weight. See and sense your lungs expanding and filling with white light as you find your breathing becoming easy and flowing. Then open your eyes.

---

Some may argue that this is "only imagination" and therefore it can't solve Cheryl's problems with the asthma, her memories of the abuse, and her difficulty in moving forward in her life. But it is imagination, not repetitive discussion and logical analysis of your story (or experience) that permits you to discover those beliefs that underlie your difficulty. By using imagery to focus on your beliefs, you go from AM to FM as if you were switching a radio dial, thus expanding your range and cutting out the static that interferes when you try to break an old habit. Your image transforms your belief from an invisible saboteur into something concrete—a *visual* form (instead of a *thought* form) that can be dealt with, changed, or even eliminated. For instance, your belief that you cannot control your anger might look like the molten lava of a volcano or a rampaging tiger. By seeing your belief as an image and then by changing this image, you are also changing the belief. We call this process "Seeing Is *Beliefing*."

---

## SEEING IS *BELIEFING*

*Intention:* To change a belief.

   *Frequency:* Use for 21 days, or whenever needed.

   Close your eyes and breathe out three times. See your belief take on an image form—for example, anger becomes lava or a rampaging tiger. Change this image if you want—the lava cascades into the sea, you do something to calm the tiger. See the new image that appears—a cool green mist, a playful kitten.

   Notice how you feel and what happens when you do this.

---

Conventional psychology adheres to the theory that it's our past experiences—our upbringing, our parents—that define who we are, what we believe, and what is or is not possible for us. But this work, which is informed by a psycho-*spiritual* rather than a psycho-*logical* perspective, teaches that it is our *beliefs* that generate our experiences in life and that once we become aware of these beliefs, they cease being invisible and we have the option of changing them and setting ourselves free.

When Cheryl practiced the imagery exercise, which took her only a minute, it gave her renewed energy and strength to go forward in life after being stuck for several years. Though she could not change the actual experiences of her past, she *could* change her attitudes, beliefs, and feelings toward them. Imagining Grandma as strong instead of weak gave Cheryl an imagery mantra she could then use to generate new actions in what had previously been difficult situations. Now, when Mom becomes abusive and tries to steamroll her, instead of having an outburst or suppressing her anger, Cheryl can employ the image of Grandma picking Mom up by her neck and carrying her off. This adds a touch of lightness and humor; it reminds Cheryl that her grandmother still watches over her and that her mom is not as powerful or unmanageable as she had previously believed.

In addition, the imagery supports Cheryl in breaking her habit (and Grandma's habit before her) of allowing her mother to get away with being a mean-spirited presence pressing her down, restricting her breath, and limiting her life. In doing this, she corrects this family error for herself and sets an example for the rest of the family as well.

## ANGELS AND IMAGERY

Cheryl's imagery experience in which an angelic presence appears is not uncommon. In the Western spiritual tradition, angels play an important part as messengers of God. Over the past few years more and more books have appeared describing experiences that people have had with angels in their everyday lives. Whether or not you believe in angels or in God, images of these spiritual beings may unexpectedly appear in your imagery and dreams. If this occurs, you then have the opportunity to explore or ignore them. Should you find yourself making negative judgments about the value of such an experience, remember that this is a judgment and is not necessarily the "truth."

## MEET THE COMMITTEE

The Judge (the part of you that makes the kind of judgment we just mentioned) is a member of what we call *the Committee*.[9] This board of directors, which lives in your head, is known also as the *false selves* or *false voices*. Once you begin to second-guess yourself and become concerned with gaining outside acceptance and approval, it's easy to fall under their spell. The members of the Committee dedicate themselves throughout your lifetime to keeping you stuck in your old habits and beliefs. They preach doom and gloom at every turn. One of their favorite ploys is demanding proof: "Just show me an angel, any angel at all. Get one in the room now and I'll believe you!" Another is playing the skeptic: "Who do you think you're kidding? Come on, that will never work." Committee members have a vested interest in retaining the status quo. When threatened, they try their best to keep things from changing.

We all fear the unknown and try to avoid discomfort; our Committee members are no different. Who would we be if we were not our old, familiar selves? The Committee member called the Skeptic constantly doubts the value of things that seem unfamiliar. If you react in a negative way to the idea of the Committee, or if you doubt that any of this could be useful for treating asthma, you can be sure it's your Skeptic planting seeds of doubt to prevent you from straying into unknown territory. After all, who knows what mischief you might get into out there?

Keeping in mind that the Committee may have various opinions about angels, let's hear about a visit from a guardian angel.

## A Visit from an Angel

John Carroll, a forty-nine-year-old businessman from Woodstock, New York,[10] had been severely allergic and asthmatic for twenty years. What began as a reaction to a cat six months later became an allergy to all household animals and soon grew to include grasses, trees, mites, molds, feathers, and several foods. For eighteen years these allergies got progressively worse. John went from taking one allergy shot every three weeks to taking two shots in a single week, using nasal steroid sprays every hour, taking an assortment of antihistamines, and spending a hundred fifty dollars on vitamin supplements a month. By 1994, John could no longer make a simple social visit to friends. Just standing near someone who was wearing a down jacket would trigger an allergic reaction.

While attending a weekend workshop on spiritual medicine at the Pathworks Center in Phoenicia, New York, John's life took a sudden turn. As he practiced some imagery he had been given, his guardian angel appeared before him looking very depressed. After his initial surprise, John realized that for years he had been ignoring this special and valuable part of himself, which he described as his "connection to spirit." He promised himself and his angel he would never do this again. A few days later the image of the angel re-appeared, only now its sadness had been transformed to joyfulness and it was blowing a trumpet. "I smiled," John said as he recounted his experience, "because I knew that after all this time, we were finally reconnected."

The following day he had another imagery experience that involved *decreating* (imaginally rooting out) a belief about an allergy he had to pizza. When he looked inside himself via his imagery, he saw the face of his ex-wife; when he removed her he felt relieved and free. Later the same day he went and had pizza. Nothing happened. The allergic, asthmatic symptoms had vanished. After these two imagery experiences the asthma stopped, and John has gone on to make this practice part of his daily life, both personally and professionally.

Over the years, many clients have told us of the presence of angels and other spiritual encounters in their imagery and dreams. This particular aspect of imagery is something that may or may not interest you. Yet the option to explore it always remains open.

## ENTERING THE "INVISIBLE WORLD"

When you begin to practice imagery, you go beyond the everyday world of material objects, linear time, and three-dimensional space and enter the invisible world. The invisible world does not contradict the visible but is rather its secret counterpart—a world of timelessness, intuition, imagination, and dreams, a world without material substance, where the extraordinary and unexpected is the rule, not the exception.[11] We've all had a taste of this invisible world: an idea or a solution to a problem that has been troubling us comes to us in a dream; the phone rings and we intuitively know who it is, even though we may not have heard from that person for months or even years; we pray or wish for something and it comes true; someone close to us becomes ill and suddenly there's a spontaneous healing; we feel a sense of foreboding and discover that a friend or a relative has been injured or died. Many people label this type of experience random, just a meaningless coincidence. Yet, by doing so, they miss out on a large part of life where, if only for a moment, we are able to connect with our innate power and creativity.

The everyday, material world is more familiar. It abides by the laws of physics and the parameters of daily life. Gravity keeps us earthbound. We plan our schedules to get places at a certain time. We work to achieve goals and measure our rewards in terms of what we accomplish, how much we have, and how pleasurable life may be. We expect things to function in a certain way. Sometimes they do. When they don't, we become frustrated and search for reassurance. But rather than perceiving these worlds as good or bad, we would better serve ourselves by recognizing how they complement each other and provide us with a balance that otherwise could not exist.

It's in the invisible world, where all is possible, that we have the opportunity to discover and explore our unique blueprint, a design or imprint that reveals the essence of our nature along with the meaning and purpose of our lives. Your blueprint is not an iron-clad list of rules and predictions. It's your own North Star—a personal compass for keeping yourself on course. When we live according to this blueprint, we walk to the beat of our own drummer instead of measuring ourselves against the standards and expectations of others. This results in a sense of health and well-being. And should physical symptoms appear, whether asthmatic or any other, we recognize them as indicators that we have somehow compromised our integrity and violated our blueprint.

These invisible and visible realities together form our entire universe; one cannot exist without the other.[12] The chart below shows how the elements that compose the everyday world, represented by the horizontal axis, have their counterpart in the invisible world, represented by the vertical axis.[13]

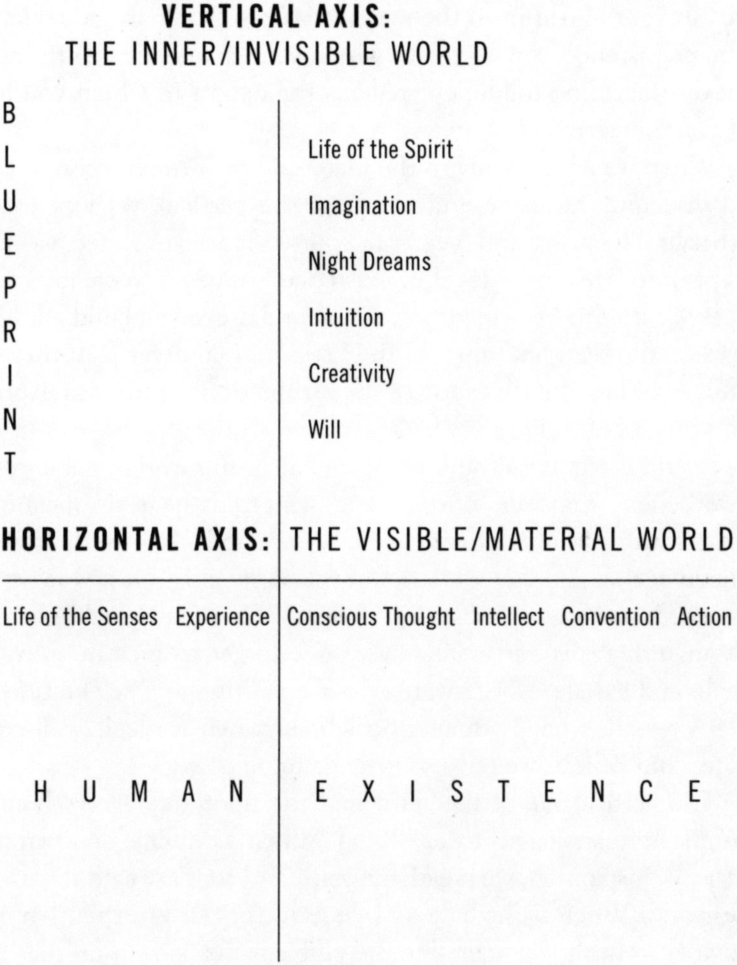

**VERTICAL AXIS:**
**THE INNER/INVISIBLE WORLD**

B
L      Life of the Spirit
U
E      Imagination
P
R      Night Dreams
I
     Intuition
N
T      Creativity

     Will

**HORIZONTAL AXIS:** THE VISIBLE/MATERIAL WORLD

Life of the Senses   Experience | Conscious Thought   Intellect   Convention   Action

H U M A N     E X I S T E N C E

Figure 4.1

As the chart illustrates, the blueprint is your personal reference point for all the elements of the invisible world: the life of the spirit connects you to God or your Higher Power; imagination is the language in which the blueprint was written; your night dreams show you how closely you are following it; and intuition flourishes as a result of living it out. The inspiration that comes of living your blueprint sparks creativity, and will is the force that you exert to live out your blueprint in the material world. While in the realm of human existence, the degree to which you experience health, happiness, peace, and fulfillment reflects the extent to which you live out your blueprint in everyday life.

When we adhere only to the material life of the horizontal axis and discount the value and power of the vertical, we lose touch with our blueprint and veer off course. However, once we pay attention to this other level of existence, we begin to create a balance. We do this by using imagination and dreams to build a bridge between the seen and unseen, the horizontal and vertical, thereby finally enabling ourselves to see the asthmatic symptoms as expressions of our entire life story.

Breath is life. If we think we wound up in this world by chance— if we believe that our suffering and symptoms have no meaning, that the world is chaotic, that who we are and what we do, think, believe, feel, and dream does not affect our health—it will leave us depressed, powerless, isolated, and numb. Eventually such existential anguish takes our breath away. We forget to breathe fully, to inhale and exhale, to be aware of our breathing as a celebration of life. After all, what is there to celebrate when we feel so disconnected and believe we have so little genuine power?

The vertical life of the spirit and the horizontal life of human existence are analogous to breathing. When we inhale and perform the act of inspiration, we breathe in spirit and connect with the invisible world. When we exhale and perform the act of expiration, we activate our healing potential in the visible world of everyday life.

Physical and environmental causes alone do not explain why the incidence of asthma has increased. The deeper source is an intense spiritual malaise—a feeling of loss, a lack of genuine connection and joy. We have become unbalanced, weighed down by the seductive promises of material life. This avid pursuit of things outside ourselves, including possessions, power, and status, has left us literally breathless and depressed. We have forgotten the invisible reality that is our source and our redemption.

As you have already begun to see, through the use of imagination and the practice of imagery, we can address this forgetting and begin to redeem ourselves. Imagery returns us to our senses and fosters real relationships with ourselves, others, and the world. Simple to learn, this type of mental work takes only a few minutes to do, and can be done anywhere, anytime. The following guidelines are a way of recalling what you have learned thus far.

## THE PRACTICAL PRACTICE OF IMAGERY:
## THREE ESSENTIAL GUIDELINES

*Commit to a daily practice.* Imagery is mind medicine in its most potent form. For conventional medication to work, you must take it regularly, for a prescribed length of time. With imagery you must do the same. Sometimes that means you practice two or three times a day, sometimes once, and at other times whenever necessary for a certain number of days. However, one of the greatest advantages of imagery is that you don't need to worry about overdosing or side effects. It's nontoxic and nonaddictive. If you do neglect the work, it's likely that the Judge or the Critic will try to engage you in a dialogue about how inadequate, bad, or forgetful you are and why your behavior is "wrong." This is a typical Committee harangue that ends up going nowhere, at least nowhere that's good for you. All you need do is acknowledge your error (yes, we all do make them), forgive yourself on the spot, and then return to the process without getting caught up in the Committee's criticism.

*Know your intention.* What do you want to change, do, accomplish, let go of, learn, heal, find? For example, you may want to heal yourself of asthma, reduce its symptoms, handle a relationship differently, or leave a stressful job. Once you know what you want, set your intention, without concern for the outcome. This means you actively stop yourself from creating "stories" about the future—about what will be, could, should, might, or might not be. This insidious practice of the Committee plants seeds of doubt, sets up expectations, and prevents your living in the present moment. Keep your inner eye here, not there, firmly rooted in the now—and like a farmer planting the seed for a healthy crop, do what is necessary to cultivate its growth. Don't dig up the new fruits each day to see what's going on with them. If you wait patiently until the seeds ripen, they come forth on their own.

*Keep this work to yourself* and trust your imagery to lead you. Don't discuss or analyze the content of your imagery. If you tell others, even those closest to you, the details of what you are doing, they invariably will react. Since we are all suggestible, you need to keep your mind free from outside comments and unsolicited advice. Remember, when you start talking, thinking, or judging, the imagery stops and the Committee takes over. Your images are your truth. Learning to trust this truth instead of running to others for approval and acceptance is the same as learning to trust yourself, which is an essential part of all healing. Once you have seen imagery's powerful effects, you can then begin to share your successful experience with others.

By doing this work you will be able to identify and address the emotions, beliefs, and social interactions that relate to your illness and affect your health. Even if you think your disease is different in its severity or nature from what others experience—that what you believe, think, and feel has no impact on your symptoms—you have nothing to lose by working with this process. What you may gain, however, is invaluable: your freedom to breathe and your ability to live an active and joyful life.

### CHAPTER 5

# THE ROAD TO RECOVERY

## An Introduction to the FUN Program

*There ain't much fun in medicine, but there's a heck of a lot of medicine in fun.*

JOSH BILLINGS

What could be fun about asthma? Finding it hard to breathe is certainly nothing to laugh at. Perhaps you feel offended or even shocked by our putting together "fun" and "asthma." Asthma is a life-threatening and debilitating disease, and we do not mean to trivialize its importance. However, we *have* found that the FUN approach can be a powerful and effective antidote. And in light of this we have chosen it as the foundation of our mindbody healing system.

## THE ESSENTIALS OF HAVING **FUN**

Fun is a way of life; it's light and lighthearted. It's the opposite of heavy and serious. Fun is the attitude that Norman Cousins, author of *Anatomy of an Illness,* used to heal himself of a disease that his doctors had said was irreversible. Fun is embodied in our having a sense of humor about life's disappointments, our losses, our pain, our errors, ourselves. Fun is a natural, organic part of life that many of us have forgotten. Except for children. For kids even crossing the street, going to the grocery store, or eating an ice cream cone can be fun. As adults we tend to lose this natural sense of enjoyment. Our fun depends on our circumstances. When our lives become painful, we tend to hold onto the pain and embody it. We feel tense, stressed out, overburdened. Our response is to tighten our muscles, to forgo smiles and laughter, to take life very seriously. And eventually this manifests as illness.

Fun, humor, and laughter provide the freedom from seriousness that is essential to living asthma free. The symptoms of asthma are the opposite of fun in every way. Instead of opening you up, loosening the muscles, relaxing you, asthma narrows you down, constricts, stresses you out. Joy opens the heart and the lungs, just as fear and rancor close and block them. Fun, humor, laughter, and joy create a pause in our suffering, transform it, and give us the room to relax and to breathe. Your Committee members will deny this to their last breath, but even in the throes of an asthma attack, shifting your perspective, taking time out from the debilitating beliefs you hold about what *may* happen, and smiling instead of frowning can relax your facial, neck, chest, back, and stomach muscles. This allows you to break the cycle of tension and fear and, in turn, can relieve the symptoms. Do we mean that you should ignore your symptoms as you gasp for breath? Of course not. What it does mean is that you take time out to see the asthma in a new light, one in which you set aside your prejudices and preconceived ideas about illness.

This, in essence, is the FUN approach: to Focus on the asthma in a new way; to Undo (reverse, eliminate) old patterns of thought and behavior; and to Now Act so as to transform those life situations that suppress and suffocate you. We do not ask that you immediately adopt this way of thinking just on our say-so. Neither do we intend to deny your pain. But we do suggest that as you read about others who have used this successfully, and as you practice the exercises throughout this book you will discover how the FUN program offers a comprehensive solution to the complex problem of asthma. Through the following story, Kathy relates how FUN first became important to her.

## TUNING IN TO BODY LANGUAGE AND BELIEFS

In 1981, I moved from Toledo, Ohio, to New York City, and my health flourished. At the time, I thought this was because I was surrounded with concrete instead of grass and flowers. After meeting a man and falling in love, I uprooted myself and moved to Florida to be with him, and the asthma returned. This time I assumed it was the dampness and vegetation that did it. Again I had focused on the outside circumstances. Trying to ferret out the reasons for my sudden relapse by paying attention to my outer environment seemed a logical way to go. My doctors never questioned me about what was going on in my emotional life, and they, after all, were the experts, so I ignored my body's message.

If I had tuned in to what was going on emotionally and mentally, I might have noticed that in leaving my hometown, I had also left behind a restricting relationship with my family, especially with my mother. At the time I thought it just a fortunate coincidence that in New York I breathed more freely and felt lighter, happier, more spontaneous. I neglected to consider that the restrictions I felt—first with my mother, who believed she knew what was best for me, and then with my lover, who insisted he knew what was best for the both of us—might be an important part of this recurring disease.

One day, during a severe attack, I automatically reached for my inhaler. Yet the medication did me no good. I immediately sensed that this wasn't the answer, not anymore. The attack reminded me that I was suffocating in more ways than one. My belief in a solution that would allow me to have it all (both the lover who insisted on holding me so close that I couldn't breathe and the freedom necessary for me to thrive as an autonomous, healthy human being) had come home to roost. I had been holding my breath, literally and figuratively, while hoping the pieces of my life would fall into place. But the tight feeling in my chest mirrored my error in thinking, and my breathing got even worse. I was stuck, clinging to an old belief about the way things *should* be. However, my body was speaking to me, loud and clear! It forced me to see that what I believed, thought, and felt was a double-edged sword. It could continue to tear me apart, or, if I would only release my beliefs along with my breath, it could provide me with emotional and physical strength. It was this realization that opened the door to a kind of healing that none of my doctors had ever suggested was possible.

Oddly enough, it was my pain that inspired me. The word *inspiration* means the act of drawing air into the lungs, while in another sense it's defined as the taking in of spirit.[1] Since I was living a life of emotional suffocation that cut off the flow of both these elements, it was no coincidence that my physical symptoms and smothering circumstances arose together. To heal, I had to reverse and release the emotional patterns, the limiting beliefs, and the twisted values that were smothering me.

## THE 180-DEGREE AHA: HAVING **FUN**!

When I first recognized that my symptoms and pain were important spiritual glyphs (or signs), I had a physical and mental "Aha." Finally I realized that the key to my healing lay, not in the neverending story about the way my life *should* be (romantically coupled, well ordered, professionally successful, dutiful, and so forth), but in having FUN. Fun was (and still remains) something I need in my everyday life to keep myself balanced and breathing freely. In truth, fun is even more than that. It's a way of being in life—living it joyfully. Writer Marilyn Ferguson describes fun as "joy in action."[2] We, the authors, thoroughly agree, and we've taken it even further. In this program FUN stands for:

# FOCUS

Focusing is a wake-up call, a type of thinking that is both energizing and relaxing. You pay attention nonjudgmentally to what goes on in life. You become a watcher. This includes looking at symptoms, beliefs, relationships, and circumstances without having your Committee dictate what is good or bad, right or wrong, normal or abnormal. When you Focus you give yourself the space to take a breath. This alone can make a physical shift occur.

# UNDO

Undoing is a reversing process. After Focusing (or watching), you choose what you want to Undo (change, eliminate, get rid of). If you use a computer, you are familiar with the Undo icon. Click on this icon, and you Undo any errors you may have made in your work. Here, we show you how to use *mind* technology to Undo, or reverse, whatever difficulties may be going on in your life. Difficulties with asthma symptoms, beliefs, relationships, and circumstances can all be undone with this process.

# NOW ACT

Action is paramount to making a healing turn. No matter what you learn, if you don't act on it in your daily life, it just sits there without doing you much good. The Now Act part of the FUN acronym helps you realize the healing potential of both Focusing and Undoing through detailed suggestions for knowing what to do and getting yourself to do it. If you tend to procrastinate, this section will help you get beyond this habit and move on with your healing and your life.

These three steps—Focus, Undo, and Now Act—form the three essential movements of mindbody healing work. First, one must *recognize* the issue. To do this requires a moment of stepping away from the emotional story or the physical symptom; you cannot see the painting or understand its meaning if you stand pressed up against it. Second, you need to *reverse* the situation and experience how it would be to live without turmoil; even if you imagine this for only an instant, it allows you an expanded glimpse of life. Third, you must *now act*; you must bring this new perspective into your current, everyday existence and not confine it to intellectual awareness.

These healing directions are valuable links that we find missing from conventional treatment. While allopathic medicine concentrates on the physiology of this disease, the bodily symptoms, and the pharmacological solutions, it brings only temporary relief. By offering us no way to synthesize our life experience with the illness, it encourages us to regard asthma as a separate event—one that has little or nothing to do with who we are and how we relate to the world.

## FINDING FREEDOM

Asthma, however, is more than an isolated event—if we want to heal ourselves, we must find a way to make sense of an illness that we are taught to believe is random and unfair. From the mindbody perspective, asthma is a crucial reminder. It tells us that we have neglected essential parts of our being—that we are living according to standards that do not match our unique blueprint, our personal truth.

Your Committee, those false selves that resist change and demand proof, want no part of this blueprint. They may well interfere, getting you stuck in internal dialogue such as "Let's see, do I really believe that? And if I don't, why should I be doing these exercises?" These seeds of doubt can be distracting. But as you get to know your Committee you will find that the more it protests something's existence and value, the more certain you can be that it's acting in its own best interests, not yours.

Losing touch with your blueprint is analogous to losing touch with your personal nature or truth. This leads to falling into a dark hole sometimes described as depression, anxiety, and emotional or physical illness. The following poem sheds light on what happens when this occurs. It's called "Autobiography in Five Chapters."[3]

1) I walk down the street.
There's a deep hole in the sidewalk.
I fall in.
I am lost . . . I am hopeless.
It isn't my fault.
It takes me forever to find a way out.

2) I walk down the same street.
There is a deep hole in the sidewalk.
I pretend I don't see it.
I fall in again.
I can't believe I'm in the same place.
But it isn't my fault.
It still takes a long time to get out.

3) I walk down the same street.
There is a deep hole in the sidewalk
I see it is there.
I still fall in . . . it's a habit
My eyes are open
I know where I am
It is my fault.
I get out immediately.

4) I walk down the same street.
There is a deep hole in the sidewalk.
I walk around it.

5) I walk down another street.

The main issues addressed in the FUN program lead to a comprehensive healing and are mirrored by this simple poem. They include: attachment, loss, truth, personal responsibility, change, and freedom. Take a few moments now and look back over the poem. See where these issues arise, and how they are resolved through using the elements of FUN. Notice how the healing process is ongoing, a continuum that begins with the pain of attachment to a victimized view of life ("I fall into the hole, and it's not my fault"). Yet when the light of truth begins to shine and responsibility is owned in the third stanza ("It's a habit; I know where I am; I get right out"), a change quickly ensues.

Freedom is the end result of being willing to Focus, Undo, and Now Act. First, you Focus by paying attention nonjudgmentally to the attachment and pain, the loss and refusal to take responsibility ("I am lost . . . I am hopeless; it isn't my fault"). Then you Undo by acknowledging personal responsibility and reversing your belief and experience ("I see it is there. I still fall in . . . it's a habit. My eyes are open," but "I know where I am" and "It is my fault"); and finally, you Now Act by engaging in movement to make the healing turn ("I get out immediately. I walk around the hole." Then, at last, after falling in once again, "I walk down another street").

Most of us say we want freedom in our lives—from unhappiness, stress, illness, pain—but what are we willing to release, be responsible for, and change within ourselves in order to get it? What does freedom mean to you? Think about it for a moment. You're worth it! Then do the next exercise.

## THE FREEDOM EXERCISE

*Intention:* To experience freedom.

*Frequency:* Use for up to one minute, once a day for seven days.

Close your eyes and breathe out three times.

Imagine Freedom.

See yourself being totally free.

Where are you? How do you look and feel?

What happens? Breathe out and open your eyes.

Freedom is essential to healing. What can we do to help this along? What does this involve in our everyday lives? Family therapist and author Virginia Satir describes what she calls the "Five Freedoms" in her book *Making Contact* as the following:[4]

*The Five Freedoms*
1. The freedom to see and hear what *is* here instead of what should be, was, or will be
2. The freedom to say what one feels and thinks, instead of what one should
3. The freedom to feel what one feels instead of what one ought
4. The freedom to ask for what one wants instead of always waiting for permission
5. The freedom to take risks on one's own behalf instead of choosing to be only "secure" and not rocking the boat.

The Committee cannot tolerate these freedoms. When you abide by them, it's *they* who can't breathe. They whine, complain, and tell you you're crazy. When any difficulty arises they insist it's a direct result of this type of thinking. Do not succumb to their tirades. Remember, the more they holler, the better you are doing.

The following story about Linda, an asthmatic client, illustrates how you can transcend and transform limiting, long-held beliefs and thinking, pull yourself out of even the deepest hole, and find a new street down which you may walk.

## THE TALE OF THE "GOOD GIRL"

Linda lost her mother when she was eight and her father by the time she was ten. Growing up, she lived with various relatives, always believing she needed to be a "good girl" at every moment—that if she slipped up and somehow displeased them she would be cast out and lose her already tenuous place in the world. Though she had been raised Jewish, Linda began attending Catholic school when she went to live with some distant cousins. At the age of twelve, she made her first communion and at about the same time suffered her first asthma attack. That her asthma kicked in when she had just formalized her faith in a religion in which she felt out of place is a mindbody event, not a coincidence. The asthma was a mirror of her grief. It's not surprising she lost her breath when she not only had lost her parents but also had forfeited an essential part of her background. Dr. Gerald Epstein advises that breath, as life, "is the physical equivalent of *faith*. When there are breathing problems, there's a break in living and faith as well."[5]

Linda began the program when she was sixty years old. She was a nutritional therapist who had been married and divorced and had raised children, yet she was still enslaved to the image of the good girl. During her first session she spoke so softly it was difficult to hear her without leaning forward. She had no freedom to say what she felt and thought. The good girl part of her was too concerned about saying what she ought and doing the acceptable (or right) thing; thus she spoke very quietly, just in case.

Linda first integrated the FUN approach into her daily life by Focusing on her symptoms. Beyond addressing the physical discomfort, she wanted to understand their significance. She used the image of "Taking a Weight off Your Chest." Within a week, the exercise became easier for her to do, and she was able to exhale more fully. She noticed that overall her breathing had changed for the better—that her habit of holding her breath had lessened considerably. Things were happening in other areas of her life as well, where she had begun to Focus on questions and issues that for fifty years had remained buried inside her.

Within a short time of having started the program, Linda described a dream where she saw a wolf with yellow eyes that changed into a man. "I felt a ripple throughout my body," she said, her voice filled with excitement, "and then I heard myself yell out: Now I know what magic is—it's part of the other dimension!" Linda said that the dream made her feel powerful, awake, and in touch with the part of herself from which she separated at ten when she became so good and so invisible.

The transformation of the wolf into a man mirrored a transformation within herself. Yelling out in her dream was an awakening, a reentry into life, a breakthrough. It was the opposite of her habitual demeanor. She had finally voiced a-loud her discovery and belief in the magic that was part of both herself and the invisible world—the *other dimension*. That she experienced this for the first time in a dream made it no less important; its vivid imprint served as a reminder of her emerging power. When, only a few weeks later, Linda was suddenly fired from a position at a prestigious medical institution where she had been caught in some bureaucratic backfire, she had the opportunity to live out in her everyday life what she had learned in her dream. This crisis presented her with the opportunity for transformation. Initially, the shock filled her with doubt about her worth, abilities, and performance. But instead of quietly burying these feelings alongside her other memories of loss and separation, she used the program to Focus on them nonjudgmentally. Then, through working with her dreams and imagery, she began to Undo them.

## WHEN "THE WORST" HAPPENS

For Linda, the worst had happened. She had been cast out. Yet, amazingly, life went on. She remained alive, well, and more awake than she could remember. Though at first she fell into the hole of disappointment, anxiety, and self-deprecation, she soon saw where she was and what she had forgotten (her pain was valuable), and she took responsibility for pulling herself out. Her breathing did not revert to the way it had been before she began the work. In fact, she felt as though she had let out a giant exhalation, a sigh of relief. During the past several months she had been feeling tied down at her job, and though she had known it was time for her to leave, the "good girl" had found it impossible to let go. As she continued to Focus on the misfortune of being fired, she began to see that what had initially seemed like a whack in the head had been, in effect, a spiritual emergency—a reminder of her blueprint and a key to freedom, should she choose to use it.

Being let go at work reminded Linda of her need to move forward in her life, to release the past and the good girl image—to stop holding back her emotions and her breath. She used this experience as a wake-up call to:

1. Reverse her habit of procrastination
2. Accept change more easily
3. Seize the present moment for taking action (instead of dwelling in the past)

Linda used the FUN program to Focus, Undo, and Now Act and was able to perceive this event differently. She Focused, without judgment, on her "loss." She Undid her habitual procrastination and sadness. Then she Now Acted through using the shock to wake herself up and pull herself out of the hole. When she chose to see her so-called misfortune in a different light, it became a turning point. It took on the form of a new street that she was free to walk down, now that she had noticed it was there. Though the experience was stressful, her response was empowering and served to improve her breathing, not worsen it. Indeed, it helped her return to her healing path, freeing not only her breathing but also her beliefs about what was possible.

Even if you've been walking down the same street all your life, it's never too late to wake up and break your habit. FUN enables you to let go of the victim mentality, the one that says "I have no control over this: I am helpless, hopeless, and enslaved." Instead, you become able to see the connections between disease and stress, emotions and symptoms, responsibility and freedom. By Focusing on whatever is going on in your life, Undoing your errors, and Now Acting on what needs to be changed, you become your own authority. Once we make this shift, the world around us shifts as well. The experts assume a different place. They are no longer above us while we wait below for them to tell us what's right or wrong, good or bad, normal or abnormal. We discover that when people, no matter how brilliant, powerful, or well informed, say "Jump!" we don't need to ask "How high?" We decide for ourselves what's valuable. And then we are able to choose from a far broader range of options.

If you are willing to see how you get stuck in your own life as the process of falling into the hole, you can make excellent use of it. This image (and the concurrent feelings of being lost, hopeless, and unable to find a way out) is familiar to most of us. One way to handle this would be through imagery. Simply see yourself in the hole, since having an asthma attack can feel like being enclosed in a dark space, being constricted, in pain, a victim. Then use your imagination to get yourself out; and see what happens and how you feel.

## GRIST FOR THE MILL

When FUN becomes a part of our everyday life, we open up to options we may never have noticed in the past. Whatever happens becomes grist for the mill—something to learn from, to create with, instead of something to complain about. Linda used the experience of being cast out from her workplace to begin exorcising the good girl image that had restricted her most of her life. You too can take what is difficult and use it to create a turn.

Expanding our view of ourselves and the world is liberating. Using the FUN program helps us do that. FUN offers a different way of knowing ourselves and of relating to our lives and our difficulties. Essentially, it reawakens our power to tap into the invisible as well as visible worlds. Ultimately, this enriches and heals our lives. Instead of the symptoms being the enemy, they become mirrors, barometers of our inner lives, and compasses for our return to health.

## DECIPHERING ASTHMA SYMPTOMS CAN BE **FUN**

As we Focus on asthma and its symptoms, we learn that it's not only a disease; it's a question that asks "what's the point?" It seeks to inform us of our deepest intention—an intention we have not yet integrated into our lives. The next exercise will show you how to read the messages conveyed by asthma symptoms. It gives you a FUN technique that allows you to perceive them in a new way. Without pathologizing or psychologizing your symptoms, the technique that follows offers a way to create a turn of mind where shame, blame, and guilt play no part. The meaning and purpose of the symptom are not sought through digging up stuff from the past or blaming others; they are encoded in the symptom itself.

### Tips on Deciphering the Symptom

Deciphering the symptom's message is like breaking a cryptic code. One way to decode the message is to pay attention to the etymology of the word that describes the symptom. For example, to *wheeze* comes from the Latin root meaning "to lament" and from the Old Norse meaning "to hiss." While the Latin emphasizes sadness and grief, the Old Norse suggests anger. Questions that stem from the etymology of the symptoms are questions like "What am I grieving?" or "Who, or what, am I angry with?" These questions are worlds away from asking "Why is this happening?" or the old standard "Why me?" Through asking these new questions, you may develop a different relationship with the asthma and begin to live life without being enslaved to it.

The Decoding Exercise draws from two sources: the meanings and etymologies found in *Webster's New World College Dictionary* and from everyday, idiomatic expressions. You might also want to create some of your own questions. Yours will be as legitimate as the ones written here. See which questions push a button, ring a bell, get you going, upset you, annoy you, make you *hold your breath*. Pay attention to how your body feels. Then write (or draw) anything that seems important or interesting.

---

## SYMPTOM DECODING

*Intention:* To relate your symptoms to your life and to clarify what they are telling you. As you do this, instead of allowing the Judge or Skeptic to take over, have FUN with the process.

*Frequency:* Use this whenever you want to delve into the deeper meaning of your symptoms.

*Focus on the questions.* Don't analyze or evaluate. Just answer with whatever comes to you.

*Undo your resistance.* If you feel uptight, breathe out, dismiss the Committee, do a couple of stretches, and loosen up.

*Now Act.* Write down or draw whatever comes to you without judging it. If a question sets off a bodily sensation, a series of thoughts, or the memory of a painful experience, though your Committee may demand that you run fast in the opposite direction, turn *toward,* not away, from it and write about it more fully. Turning toward the discomfort is an indispensable part of healing. You may even notice an immediate shift in any breathing difficulty you may be having when you do this.

## Wheezing
What loss am I grieving?
What am I feeling sad about?
Who or what am I angry with?

## Coughing
Who or what do I need/want to expel?
Who or what is irritating me?
What or who am I reluctant to give up?
What do I feel pressed to cough up, cough over?
What do I need to confess?

## Constriction
What or who is constricting me?
How am I constricting myself?
What in my life is coming apart?
What am I trying to hold/keep together?

## Suffocation
What am I not saying that wants or needs to be said?
Who or what is suffocating me?
Who or what am I not letting go of?

## Choking
What or who makes me feel choked up?
Who or what is holding me back (how am I feeling choked off)?
What or who am I choking on?
What do I need to say?

Pause here and reflect on these questions. Once you have worked with this exercise you may discover some powerful truths regarding your asthma symptoms. However, do not dwell on them. Put them aside and give yourself some space. As you go on, you will acquire more tools for working with these. For now this is enough.

# TRANSFORMING DISEASE AND
# DESPAIR INTO HOPE

When we refuse to pay attention to our symptoms, we reduce the disease to a meaningless experience. This leaves us stuck in a labyrinth of isolation and despair. To find hope, we learn to live in the here and now and regard our lives as valuable even if not always pleasant. Focusing on our symptoms—really listening to what they have to say—then Undoing our beliefs about our limitations and committing ourselves to Now Act to resolve our difficulties can restore us. "When our focus is toward a principle of relatedness and oneness, and away from fragmentation and isolation, health ensues."[6]

Rebbe Nachman, the Hasidic teacher, guide, and spiritual master, shared the kind of insight and wisdom that lead to healing our sense of alienation when he said:[7]

> If you believe that you can damage, then believe that you
> can fix.
>      If you believe that you can harm, then believe that you
> can heal.

and

> Never despair! Never! It's forbidden to give up hope.

In the spirit of this advice, the next imagery exercise will help prepare you for what lies ahead.

# ROAD TO RECOVERY ✳

*Intention:* To energize and empower yourself, and to generate healing.

*Frequency:* Use every day for up to three minutes, or whenever you need to renew hope.

Close your eyes and breathe out three times.

Imagine that you are preparing for an important journey. Know that this is your journey to recovery. As you embark, see yourself crossing from one side of a bridge to the other—leaving behind all illness, doubt, guilt, and anything else you find distressing. Once you reach the other side, find a special road or path that you walk on. Now, feel the golden sun shining down upon you from the clear, blue sky above. Feel your arms become very long. Reach up and take some of the sunlight in your hands. Place this sunlight in your lungs and bronchi, or anywhere else you choose in your body, to give you energy and a sense of well-being. Continue to walk, and as you do this, sense and see yourself becoming stronger and stronger, as your breath flows easily and rhythmically through your entire body. Feel and see yourself enjoying this newfound energy while knowing you can return to this path at any time. Then breathe out and open your eyes.

## MOVING ON

In the next three chapters you will find specific suggestions, exercises, and healing stories to help integrate FUN into your own life. Important elements of the FUN program involve your willingness to:

- Recognize and separate yourself from the beliefs that have been holding you hostage

- Listen to the message your symptoms convey to your body-mind
- Break free of your enslavement to your Committee—those false selves who try to prevent change, even when it heals
- Ask yourself (and remember to answer), "How am I having FUN in my life?"

To get the most out of the program, we suggest that you take your time. Instead of giving yourself a case of mental suffocation, stop along the way and enjoy what you read. Do the exercises; don't just think about them. Allow the work to come alive for you, to become part of your life, and to open the way for authentic healing. As you embark on the road to recovery, we suggest that you take note of the next six pointers, which will help prepare you for your journey, imaginal or otherwise.

*Six Pointers for Getting Started*
1. *Get a notebook* (if you haven't already). Use it to record your dreams and thoughts. This makes it easier to do the work and keep track of your progress. Here, you may write about or draw meaningful or moving experiences you have during any of the exercises or when reading passages in the text.
2. *Write your intentions.* Do this on the first page of your notebook. Answer the question: What do I want to get (learn, know, change, heal, find) through using this program? Be as specific as you can. Know that as you go on with the work, your intentions may change. Intentions provide you with a direction. They are not the same as an agenda or goals. And they are not carved in stone.
3. *Record any experiences in your daily life that seem related to this work.* This might include events you usually call coincidences; changes in your emotional or physical state; or anything you might perceive differently in yourself or in your relationships with people around you.

4. *Record any night dreams.* Write these as soon as possible after you wake up so you don't forget them, even if they are just fragments that don't seem important. Dreams are often useful for creating personal imagery for yourself, and they may embody healing messages that our logical, ordinary minds don't come up with. There will be specific information on how to use your dreams for healing in chapters 7 and 8.

5. *Get some blank tapes.* Use these to record any of the imagery exercises. Once you are familiar with the exercise, stop using the tape. When you practice the imagery without hearing an outside voice directing you, you begin to become aware of your *inner voice.*

6. *Be consistent, and do some of this work every day.* This might involve practicing an imagery exercise, reading part of the text, writing down a dream, listening to some music, or working with any part of the FUN program that you feel drawn to. Remember, the potency of imaginal medicine depends on your using it, just as you would be expected by your doctor to use your inhaler. *Thinking* about it won't do the trick, just as *thinking* about taking your regular medication would be useless.

### CHAPTER 6

# FOCUS

## The Art of Paying Attention

*The mind of the sage, being in repose, becomes the mirror of the universe.*

CHUANG TZU

> ## FOCUS
>
> - Become a Watcher
> - Dismember the Committee
> - Placebos, Nocebos, and Beliefs
> - The Belief Inventory
> - You Are Not the Symptom
> - Drawing and Dreaming
> - Relationship as a Healing Practice

Focusing, which implements the *F* in FUN, is a pivotal technique for paying attention—one that most of us have never been taught. When you Focus, you attend to asthma in a nonjudgmental way; you expand your awareness and acknowledge the personal beliefs in which your symptoms are rooted. Thus, you begin to notice that your beliefs, symptoms, and relationships are intimately connected, to one another as well as to the various circumstances of your life. Learning to Focus is an awakening process. It enables you to see how your Committee tries to undermine your authority at every moment. The allegory that follows mirrors the simplicity and importance of Focusing.

A man who had sacrificed much and worked hard traveled a great distance to meet a spiritual master from whom he hoped to learn the secret of life. Upon being introduced, though he was overwhelmed at being in the presence of this person, he finally gained the courage to ask his question.

"I have waited many years for this," he explained, "and now that I am here there is one thing that I must know before I die: What is the secret of life?" The master was quiet for a moment and then said, "There are three things, not one. Listen closely, for I will not repeat myself. The first, is *pay attention* . . . The second, is *pay attention* . . . And the third is, *pay attention*."

If the man had come looking for anything complex or obscure, he was surely disappointed.

The secret the master shared was deceptively simple. Yet it tells us a great deal. It informs us of our need to stay awake despite the hypnotic distractions of everyday existence. As you begin to cultivate the art of paying attention through Focusing, you will learn the ancient technique of "concentrating without effort."[1] In this state of mind you suspend judgment and accept not knowing as normal rather than thinking of it as a character flaw. Thus, instead of immediately seeking the solution to the difficulty, when you Focus, you restrain your ego, become detached, and say "I don't know," without worrying about why not. But when it comes to dealing with asthma, not knowing the solution, feeling detached from the symptoms, and not worrying about the future are skills that most of us have not learned to cultivate.

## BECOME A WATCHER

Becoming the Watcher can help you do this. The Watcher is accepting instead of judgmental, analytical, or self-conscious. The Watcher Focuses by forgoing control and trying to fix things. Thus, when you become the Watcher you begin to foster forgiveness of your shortcomings. You stop dwelling on things or jumping to conclusions. The ordinary, thinking mind steps aside, and you begin to *watch*, instead of *judge*, all that occurs, both on the inside and the outside. As the Watcher, you experience a sense of freedom, perhaps for the first time, from the physical symptoms of asthma and the difficulties experienced in everyday life. No shift or change is actively sought, although changes in thinking, feeling, and living usually occur as a natural consequence.[2]

The Watcher stops, looks, and listens simultaneously, noting internal reactions and external events. It doesn't try to control what's going on, to do something, or to understand the symptom or circumstance. Its sole (and *soul*) task is watching. By becoming the Watcher, you separate from your beliefs, feelings, actions, and symptoms and align yourself with the sacredness in daily life. In doing this you make a tremendous turn, as you begin to see even the simplest, or most difficult events, including the asthma, as valuable.

When you become the Watcher you practice a spiritual union of opposites; you stand as the mediator between the eternal world of spirit and the limited world of time and space. The next exercise evokes an experience of this union. As a way of preparing to Focus, you may find the following imagery useful. It reveals where you are currently standing (or the place you are now watching from) and gives you the chance to make any change you wish in your position.

## THE EYE OF THE BEHOLDER

*Intention:* To make it easier to Focus, and to Focus clearly.

*Frequency:* To be used to begin your day, or whenever you feel overwhelmed by circumstances or symptoms.

Breathe out three times. Looking down from a bird's-eye view, see below you, on a large lawn or field, what appears to be a design or imprint of a large eye. Now see yourself standing somewhere on the same field. Note where you are standing on this field in relationship to the eye. Breathe out. Now see and feel yourself walking quickly, yet without hurrying, to the center of the eye. Stand there alert, calm, and erect, knowing that you are now in place as the Watcher. Notice how you feel. Now open your eyes.

Note any observations and feelings about this experience in your journal.

This exercise allows you to center yourself imaginally. You may also use it as a brief buffer to deal with asthma symptoms and everyday circumstances that distress you. With practice you need not even close your eyes. Just breathe out, sense yourself walking to the center of the eye, and know that you are in place as the Watcher.

## WATCHING SYMPTOMS

Wallace Ellerbroek, a psychiatrist who was previously a surgeon, has taught his patients to pay attention to the symptoms of their diseases in a similar way. In one of Ellerbroek's experiments he taught chronic acne patients to respond to any new eruptions by using nonjudgmental attention. Instead of indulging themselves in a spiral of negative emotions, they were advised to *accept* the acne. This might involve looking at themselves in the mirror and speaking to the pimple as if it were absolutely fine for it to be there. They could say something like, "Well, pimple, there you are, right where you belong at this moment in time." Thus they *Focused on the symptom with acceptance and forgiveness*, watching it without trying to control or fix it. In essence, they became Watchers.

Amazingly, several patients' acne cleared up completely, despite the fact that they had been suffering with this condition for at least fifteen years. Whereas their anxiety, resentment, and resistance had been perpetuating the symptom, once they began Focusing (watching the symptom) without hostility, they gave it the space to make a graceful exit. Of course acne is not asthma, but when you Focus on asthma symptoms, the same principles and process apply. Anything that draws us into a mindful, watchful state has the power to transform.[3]

The next time you have an asthma symptom, do as Ellerbroek's patients did, using this exercise:

## TRANSFORMING SYMPTOMS BY WATCHING

*Intention:* To pay attention to symptoms in a new way.

*Frequency:* Every day for at least seven days.

Stop any mind chatter. Focus on the symptom: watch it with no preconceived story about how awful or abnormal it is. Allow it to be there without trying to control or get rid of it.

See what happens, and make a note of your response.

## DISMEMBER THE COMMITTEE

Did your Committee members intervene while you were reading this or doing the exercise? Did they argue that you can't equate asthma with acne? Did they insist that it's impossible to observe an asthma symptom in a nonjudgmental way and that standing in the middle of an eye (even in your imagination) is silly and a waste of time? The Committee insists on masquerading as reason, logic, and good old common sense—out for your "best" interests,

of course—while striving to remain in control at all times. Committee members, like the Judge, Skeptic, Namer, Blamer, Shamer,
and Storyteller, all resist change and insist on the status quo
where they know the ropes—the ones that keep you tied up in
knots while *they* call the shots. When these saboteurs make an
appearance, they reveal themselves by their habits. These include,
but are not limited to, complaining, blaming, comparing, general-
izing, and what author Joan Borysenko calls "awfulizing." Awfulizing "escalates a situation to its worst possible conclusion." It
dwells on fantasies of worst-case scenarios, both past and future.[4]
It keeps your body-mind spinning and tense, unable to relax,
think clearly, or make decisions that help you change and grow.

When the Awfulizer puts in an appearance, it tries its best to
make everything look a lot worse. A sneeze becomes a cold; the
cold inevitably leads to the flu; and the flu, well, that could become
pneumonia before you know it. Among the worst Awfulizers today
are the pathologized labels conventional medicine uses to describe
illness, qualifying it as "chronic," "incurable," and "terminal," feed-
ing this culprit just what it needs to flourish.

Instead of taking on one of these spoilers in a futile dialogue,
resisting it, or trying to run away, it's more effective to acknowledge
its presence. See it for what it is, and quickly move on. In plain
words, become the Watcher, and Focus on it without *dwelling*. This
means, do not engage in discussion or debate about whether its predictions are right or wrong, and do not listen to its threats regarding what will happen if you refuse to knuckle under. Since the
Watcher has no emotional or mental attachment to the Committee, the Committee sees him or her as its nemesis. Within a short
time, whenever the Watcher puts in an appearance, the Committee loses interest and retires from the boardroom. This sets you free
to get on with your work, life, and healing.

When Linda, the good girl whom we met in the previous
chapter, lost her job, her Committee (the Awfulizer, Skeptic,
Judge, Doubter, and so forth) immediately assembled and began to

harangue her. Yet, despite her initially being hypnotized by its rhetoric, she quickly realized her error and began to Focus. Before, she might have lived out this experience as the habitual victim, obsessing over what she had done wrong or feeling guilty for having failed. But through Focusing, it took her only a very short time to realize she was falling into that same old hole. Instead she became the Watcher: by doing this she separated herself, first from these impostors, who so desperately wanted to capture her attention, then from what she had labeled her misfortune. In making this separation, she gave herself the room that she needed in order to breathe.

## CHOOSING YOUR INTENTIONS

Before we go further and Focus on the three major areas of symptoms, beliefs, and relationships, it's important that you choose your intentions. This means you need to decide what it is you *want*. That might involve what you want to get, learn, know, become, change, heal, find, or create through using this program. Choose up to three intentions. That's enough for now. Once you've chosen them, write these intentions down on the first page of your notebook. Refer to them once in a while as you might to a compass—to keep yourself headed in your intended direction.

All of us put our own imprint on this process. While Linda's intentions were to feel whole and at peace and to live her life passionately, yours may be more specific. You may want to reduce your medication, end a debilitating relationship, or exercise without fear of inciting an asthma attack. Use the Focusing process to do this. Become the Watcher; thus you can deter the Committee from corrupting your intentions by telling you what is or isn't possible. Your choice of intention is the first step to freedom. Do not allow the Committee to get in the way. As you go along with the work, your life and your intentions will change. Intentions are more flexible than an agenda or goals. No matter what the Committee says, you are not a failure if you modify an intention. They are meant to provide you with a direction, not to be carved in stone.


## FOCUSING ON YOUR BELIEFS

Now that you have Focused on what you want, it's time to Focus on what you *believe*. A colleague of ours once taught at a prison. She told us that the best thing about it was that unlike the people she usually works with, these men *knew* they were in jail. They were able to see and feel the bars that separated them from the world. They were forced to acknowledge the guards who governed their movements. And they realized their freedom was limited.

Her point was well taken, for we on the outside are imprisoned as well. But the bars that restrict us are invisible, constructed out of our *beliefs*, those we hold that determine how much of life is actually available to us. Therefore, if I believe that my asthma holds me hostage or that I am unlovable the way I am, it's difficult to feel free or to love life as it is. To believe that only the pleasures of life hold value is to deny that there is meaning in our difficulty and pain or that they are important for our growth and healing. Being well calls for being present, involved in all of life, not just the "good" or comfortable part. When we refuse to see our beliefs as the invisible bars of our personal prisons, we sacrifice this experience of wholeness, and our bodies suffer the consequences.

Whether we are sick or well, happy or depressed, energized or depleted depends not so much on the outer experience of life but on what we believe, think, and feel. Though many might discount this as religious or philosophical supposition, new brain-scanning techniques have proven to scientists that this is not as far-fetched as they thought. This technology shows there are biological mechanisms that can turn belief or thought into an agent of biological change in cells, tissues, and organs.[5] What was once looked at as unscientific theory is now meeting the rigors of extensive testing. Thus medical experts who previously dismissed such information are being pressed by hard scientific evidence to reverse their skepticism and reconsider their opinions.

The following imagery exercise affords you the chance to experience your willingness to leave behind your imprisoning beliefs. These beliefs may relate to asthma, work, lifestyle, or persons. Try using this exercise for yourself, and see what happens.

---

## THE PRISON CELL

*Intention:* To Focus on your willingness to break free of the self-made prison formed by the beliefs, thoughts, feelings, and relationships that limit and deplete you.

*Frequency:* Do once as an exploration in Focusing. If you find that you want to make a correction in what you see, return and make the correction in your imagination, then continue for the next seven days as an experience in personal growth.

Close your eyes. Breathe out three times. Imagine you are confined in a prison cell. What does it look like? How big is it? Where are you standing? Now find beside you a key that unlocks the door to this cell. What do you do? What happens? How do you feel?

Then breathe out, open your eyes, and return.

---

Remember, no matter what your experience is in doing this, it reveals something valuable about where you are in your life, what you believe, and the way you function. Make no judgments. Instead, Focus on this as an experience in imaginal living, where there is no good or bad, normal or abnormal.

Lee, a fifty-year-old artist who had not painted since she developed asthma at forty-three, reported that she had fixed up her cell with curtains, a lovely quilt for the bed, a carpet for the floor, and paintings to decorate the walls. She mentioned no key until she was asked about it, at which point she said, "I didn't need the key. I made myself so comfortable that I had no reason to leave." The imagery makes it clear that Lee's desire to be comfortable (which was born of her belief that discomfort is "bad" and lacks value) was more important to her than becoming free or well—that freedom and healing were too dangerous to even consider at this point. Her prison, which manifests in her life as her illness, becomes her home. She prefers to suffer the pain she's familiar with rather than risk facing the unknown. And the key becomes virtually invisible to her.

Jim, a twenty-year-old acting student with asthma, found that when he walked out of the cell, he entered a room that was as dark and closed in as the first. But instead of making a judgment that this was "bad," he saw it as analogous to how stuck he felt at that moment in his life. Jim chose to continue this exercise for the next seven days. When he reported back he described how each day the room had spontaneously grown lighter and larger and how he began to feel freer and less confined, not only in his imagery, but in his breathing and everyday life as well.

According to the Talmud, an ancient Jewish text, "We do not see things as they are. We see them as *we* are." Our beliefs are the filters through which we perceive our lives. They color all of our experiences, whether emotional, mental, or physical. They determine not only what we think of ourselves, but what we think of others. While we look through these filters our vision is limited by them. When we put them aside freedom is nearby.[6]

## PLACEBOS, NOCEBOS, AND BELIEFS

Limiting beliefs, particularly when issued as a statement of fact by an authority like your doctor (or by parents, teachers, and experts), can have what is called a *nocebo* effect. Whereas in Latin the word *placebo* means "I shall please" and involves feeling better, or healing, as a result of a treatment, procedure, or pill that is not "real," a *nocebo* involves feeling worse and becoming sicker. Both are related to the power of belief, since in each case it's your belief that acts as the catalyst.

Science has been baffled for ages by effects of placebos on patients who may not only reap the reward of a "sham" medication but who suffer its side effects as well. Currently, the placebo effect is looked at as a triumph of expectation over reality, with the expectation (or what is really a belief about the near future) producing positive biochemical results. In the same way, strong belief in danger triggers stress hormones like adrenaline. Thus science is finally acknowledging, albeit obliquely, what the sages have told us for thousands of years: it is our beliefs that create our experience of life—and it's with our thoughts we create the world.

"We are misled by dualism or the idea that mind and body are separate," says Dr. Howard Fields, a neuroscientist at the University of California at San Francisco. Fields describes a thought as "a set of neurons firing, which through complex brain wiring can activate emotional centers, pain pathways, memories, the autonomic nervous system, and other parts of the nervous system involved in producing physical sensations."[7] Therefore, according to the most advanced studies, our beliefs, which are the source of our thoughts, are not vague, meaningless events in terms of our biochemistry. In fact, they are able to change our cells and organs as definitively as a "real" medication.

Even for asthmatics, who are constantly told they can't live without consistent medication, this story holds true. When asthmatic children in Venezuela were medicated with a bronchodilator along with a sniff of vanilla, twice a day, and later were given a sniff of the vanilla alone (basically no medication at all), it increased their lung function 33 percent as much as the bronchodilator had. The scent of vanilla tapped into their belief that this was a "real" medication. Their neurons fired off the message, and the body did as it was told.[8]

## TEN NOCEBO BELIEFS ABOUT ASTHMA

Just as a positive belief can evoke healing, your Committee can have a field day with your limiting beliefs and thoughts. It thrills to generating worst-case scenarios and comparisons that reduce you to bug size. If any of the following ten beliefs have taken up residence in your head, the Committee won't hesitate to use them against you. The letters next to each belief indicate the Committee's agenda. Immediately after the list you will find a key to the code letters. Before you look at the key to find out each member's special contribution to your enslavement, think of how these ten beliefs limit your life and diminish your natural ability to heal. If you have other Committee members, add them to the list. By recognizing the Committee in this way it makes it easier to *dis*-member them.

1. I'll never be happy because I have asthma. (St, N, A)
2. I need to be perfect, and my asthma prevents that. (Cm, Cd, J)
3. Asthma makes me different, abnormal. (Cm, V, N)
4. Asthma limits where I can go and what I can do. (St, Aw, Sk)
5. I'm a burden to my family and friends because of my asthma. (St, Sh, B)
6. I have asthma because my father (mother, grandparent) has it. (B, Cd, V)
7. There's nothing I can do about this disease except take my medication. (V, Cd, N)
8. This will only get worse. (Cm, Cd, J)
9. It's better not to have sex, since it might induce an attack. (St, A, Sk)
10. Asthma will shorten my life. (St, Cd, J, et al.)

*Members of the Committee*
A: The *Awfulizer* makes everything worse than it is—*much* worse.
B: The *Blamer* blames you and others for the events and circumstances of your life.

Cd: The *Concluder* jumps to habitual and safe conclusions.

Cm: The *Comparer* elevates or devalues your worth.

J: The *Judge* judges right from wrong; good from bad; normal from abnormal.

N: The *Namer* labels people, events, and diseases.

Sh: The *Shamer* instills embarrassment, guilt, and fault.

Sk: The *Skeptic* makes you doubt your own experience.

St: The *Storyteller* comments knowingly on the future or the past.

V: The *Victimizer* makes you the injured party, by your own hand or another's.

The Storyteller says, "I'll never be happy because I have asthma." This is an evil fairy tale about the future. How do we know what will happen? The Namer labels this collection of physical sensations an illness called asthma. The Awfulizer makes the smallest sign of illness into a catastrophe, thus isolating you from a healthy and normal life. Saying "I have asthma because my father has it" is the Blamer's way of assigning responsibility to someone else. The Concluder decides that there is no escape, ever, since asthma is "genetic." This allows the Victimizer to get right to its task of insisting that you are and always will be a victim. The belief that "It's better not to have sex since it might induce an asthma attack" gives the Judge power to determine right from wrong and to limit your pleasure. The Comparer weighs the merit of your actions. The Shamer makes you feel guilty for wanting to enjoy yourself. The Skeptic believes "Asthma limits where I can go and what I can do," thus denying the possibility that you can do exactly what you want.

With the help of the Committee, these beliefs become our mental children and manipulate us with their constant demands for attention. When you Focus on and separate yourself from such beliefs, you create a space of freedom.[9] This thwarts the Committee, which counts on your enslavement to limiting beliefs for its survival.

## THE RISKS AND REWARDS OF RESPONSIBILITY

The fourth step of the twelve-step program of Alcoholics Anonymous involves doing a moral inventory, which means that you admit (and actually list) your liabilities and look squarely at the unhappiness you have created for others and yourself. The program proposes that by uncovering your "emotional deformities" [10] you move toward correcting them; without this you can't experience genuine sobriety or contentment. Even though alcoholism is considered by many to be a disease rather than just a habit, Alcoholics Anonymous advises that to reach sobriety, you must take responsibility for your illness. To do this, you first look inward to determine the beliefs, desires, and thoughts that govern your actions.

When you become addicted to the belief that your experiences are not your responsibility—that by taking responsibility you are being made to feel guilty—you are buying into a myth created by the Storyteller and the Blamer. They create this myth with the express purpose of encouraging you to hand over responsibility (and power) to someone or something else (your parents, your doctor, genetics, luck, fate, and so forth). This, in turn, makes it impossible to become your own authority or to move any closer to true freedom and to the divine source.

The Belief Inventory that follows parallels the fourth step of Alcoholics Anonymous. It's a practical method for Focusing on the beliefs by which you live your life each moment yet that most of us rarely question or even realize exist. Once you know your limiting beliefs, you can begin to Undo them. This generates a shift in your body-mind that furthers your ability to live and breathe more freely in your everyday life.

# THE BELIEF INVENTORY

In your notebook list at least one or more beliefs you hold about each of the following (you may write and/or draw a symbol for each). Though it may be difficult to state your beliefs in a few sentences, just do what you can without concern for how it sounds or if it would make sense to anyone else. Even a few words will do. The first thing that comes to you is fine. The less you deliberate, the better. You can always return and fill in the gaps.

1. Something you believe about change.
2. Something you believe about responsibility.
3. Something you believe about love.
4. Something you believe about your body.
5. Something you believe about loss.
6. Something you believe about sadness.
7. Something you believe about freedom.
8. Something you believe about your parents.
9. Something you believe about your worth.
10. Something you believe about your sexuality.
11. Something you believe about pain.
12. Something you believe about anger.
13. Something you believe about guilt.
14. Something you believe about forgiveness.
15. Something you believe about being a woman or man.
16. Something you believe about joy.
17. Something you believe about health.
18. Something you believe about asthma.

When you're done, after each belief you wrote down, note whether it is (H) helpful to you or (L) limiting to you.

# WORKING WITH YOUR BELIEFS

The beliefs in the inventory you just completed have the power to heal or harm. When talking to ourselves, even when the words are not spoken aloud, our thoughts can have a strong effect on the body. By saying, "I'm worried sick," "my heart is broken," "you're suffocating me," or the ultimate killer, "I'd rather be dead," we're constantly firing off unwitting messages that we can ill afford. In light of how our beliefs influence our experience and our lives, it's important to know not only what they are but what to do with them.

## Separating and Creating Space

Now that you have made an inventory of your beliefs, how do you work with them? Conventional psychotherapy tells us that insight will do it for us. When we know and understand the cause of our difficulty, we're supposed to be healed or at least feel somewhat better. But this provides only a brief fix. As James Hillman and Michael Ventura so aptly put it in the title of their reproach to conventional psychology: "we've had a hundred years of psychotherapy—and the world's getting worse."[11] Is it really enough just *to know* your beliefs? Is this any more likely to get you unstuck than insisting the reason for your fear of loss, separation, and death is that your mom forgot to pick you up after school one day in first grade? Knowledge of your beliefs *is* essential, but if you insist on being *attached* to that knowledge and making up stories about it, it becomes just one more obstacle that prevents you from moving on.

In *Being Peace*, the poet and Zen master Thich Nhat Hanh tells us, "If we take one thing to be the truth and cling to it, even if truth itself comes in person and knocks at our door, we won't open it. For things to reveal themselves to us, we need to be ready to abandon our views about them."[12] What is understanding? In the case of Focusing, understanding is modest, empty of ego and belief. It means "to throw away your knowledge. The technique is to *release*." Focusing allows us to do this.

In the next exercise, we introduce you to a simple process for separating from those beliefs that create limitation or illness in your life. By separating from a belief, you release yourself from its influence, which in turn allows you to eliminate or transform it. When you practice this technique, Focus rather than think. Don't try to figure it out. There is no right or wrong way, no matter what the Committee members tell you.

## SEPARATING AND CREATING SPACE

*Intention:* To detach from and release any circumstance, person, belief, or event (past or present).

*Frequency:* Use as needed.

Look around the room you are in right now, and name or identify aloud three different things that you see.

Look at the first thing. Can you *feel a separation* between yourself and whatever this is (for example: the computer, table, book)? Although the keyboard of your computer may be right beneath your fingertips, once you name or identify it as "computer" or "keyboard," you differentiate from it; that is, you know you are separate, that it is not "me."

Now *feel the space* between you and this object. If you stop and Focus, or concentrate without effort, you will begin to feel that there is definitely space between you. As you continue to Focus, you will become further and further apart and sense that there is even more space between you and the computer than you first experienced.

Now do this again with the two remaining things that you have chosen to name. Name them, one at a time. Feel the *separation* from each. Then feel *the space* separating you from the object.

Now think of a belief that's negative or limits you. Try using one of the beliefs in your Belief Inventory. Then go through the same process again. Identify or name it (belief, idea, thought). Feel a separation from it. Then create some space between you and it. What happens when you do this? Write down your response in your notebook.

If you don't separate from your belief immediately, don't be discouraged. Though most people separate from objects pretty easily, beliefs are far more tenacious. Detaching or separating from them takes practice, and using the exercise for "Becoming the Watcher" beforehand can be helpful.

## SEPARATION, LOSS, AND ASTHMA

Whatever difficulty you have in feeling this separation between yourself and your belief shows how closely you're attached to it. Attachment, separation, and loss, particularly having to do with parents, are major emotional issues for people with asthma. When asked, many asthmatics tell us that their initial diagnosis appeared around the time of parental divorces, of parents or loved ones leaving them in one way or another, or when they themselves were first leaving home. Emily, the child whose experience with asthma you will be reading about in chapter 9, had her first asthma attack at the age of three. This was shortly after her mother was diagnosed with ovarian cancer. Even though no one had discussed the possibility that her mother might die, she knew this could happen, and the thought of this separation was unbearable. It was at this time the asthma surfaced.

Bob, a twenty-eight-year-old law student, was diagnosed with asthma at thirteen, two years after his father and mother separated. He claimed that at the time he had just "gotten over being angry" with his father, whom he described as a controlling and abusive man. However, Bob's anger (which he believed he had put behind him) still pursued him in his dreams, where he often found himself fleeing from a mob of menacing, angry strangers threatening to harm him. Clearly he was right, the anger *was* behind him, but not in the way he meant. In fact, it manifested in his body, where it called out to be addressed by way of his symptoms.

When Andrea, who had been on strong psychotropic medication for several years, first did the "Separating and Creating Space" exercise, she had trouble feeling a separation, even from the chair on which she sat. It was as if she had lost all sense of her personal boundaries. By depending so thoroughly on this outside agent (the medication) to keep her going, she had handed over her authority to the experts and had lost touch with who she was. The shock of this experience brought to light a belief that she had held for as long as she remembered—one that told her she wasn't worth much. She once confided that her sister had remarked how she continually "apologized for every breath she took"—a stunning reminder that the asthma had found a perfect host.

In this section you Focused on the danger of becoming a prisoner of your limiting beliefs and learned how to use this process to separate from them. The next part of the chapter shows you how to Focus on your symptoms, thus diminishing their impact and power.

## FOCUSING ON SYMPTOMS

For an asthmatic, the most pressing question is "How do I get rid of my symptoms?" The automatic connection between the fear of not being able to breathe and not being able to live creates a palpable anxiety. Yet our insistence on eliminating this anxiety immediately by annihilating the symptom is misguided. We agree that getting rid of your symptoms is a valuable intention and an important part of this program, but your symptom is only the tip of the iceberg, an indication of something else. It's equally important, and more valuable in terms of your healing process, to learn what the symptom means within the overall context of your life. For only by turning *toward* the symptom— which also involves going through and beyond your anxiety—are you able to release it.

In the beginning of this chapter, you learned how Wallace Ellerbroek's patients used a technique similar to Focusing to watch their acne symptoms. Perhaps, as we suggested, you have already tried it yourself. You also did the exercise for making a separation and creating a space between you and your beliefs. Symptom Focusing naturally evolves from these exercises. It can be done in several ways and, of itself, often creates a marked improvement. Using the following process is a good way to begin.

---

## YOU ARE NOT THE SYMPTOM ✳

*Intention:* To separate yourself from the symptom.

*Frequency:* Whenever a symptom comes up, or as often as you can.

The next time you experience an asthma symptom, instead of reaching for your medication, stop, and close your eyes.

Now *Focus* on (just watch) the part of your body where you're feeling discomfort.

Name or *label* the symptom—wheezing, constriction, discomfort, tightness, coughing. Or just label it "symptom."

Then feel a *separation* between you and this physical symptom.

Recognize that you are not the symptom (the wheezing, coughing, constriction) by saying aloud, or in your imagination, *"I am not the symptom. I am (say your name)."*

See, sense, and feel how you now *create a space of freedom.* Then slowly open your eyes.

---

Even if you can't immediately feel a separation, stay with the symptom process for up to a minute or two. Focus without telling a story, complaining, or running away from it. Know, for now, that this is enough; the separation will come with practice. Do this without getting attached to the outcome. Soon you will find that your separation from the symptom and the genuine realization that "I am not the symptom" will arise naturally. As you practice, you begin to distance yourself from the wheezing, coughing, tightness, or heaviness, which in turn gives you a sense of empowerment, release, and relief.

## DRAWING THE SYMPTOM

Drawing the symptom is another technique for Focusing, one that is nonverbal and that can actually be FUN. It helps create a separation from the symptom by bringing the inside (your beliefs, images, feelings, sensations, and thoughts) to the outside through the drawing. This process is simple.

---

### DRAW THE SYMPTOM

*Intention:* To create a separation and space between you and the symptom.

*Frequency:* Use the process once. Then draw again in three weeks and note any changes.

Sit down with some paper and colors, then draw the symptom. When you finish, put it aside or tuck it into your notebook. That's it for now.

*Note: You could also draw the Committee. They will try to talk you out of it, but pay no attention. It's worth doing just for the FUN of it.*

---

After using the Focusing process, Nicole, whose asthmatic symptoms had recently recurred, drew a picture of her symptom. In her drawing, only the top part of her body appeared. Her breathing passages looked like tiny, narrow tubes, and she drew her lungs as shrunken and folded in on themselves. Nicole explained that drawing the symptom and seeing it on paper made her understand what her body was going through. She said it helped her to separate from the feelings of fear that made the symptom worse. "It's as if putting it *out here* gives me relief and more space to breathe *in there*," she said, first touching the paper, then her chest.

Nicole felt the image of the narrow tubes and shrunken lungs was in many ways analogous to her life. During the past two years she had experienced a narrowing down of opportunities, a shrinking of joy and pleasure. Her career as a singer, which had brought her admiration and status, came to a halt when she shifted gears and chose to go into acting instead. But the acting world refused to welcome her with open arms as she had hoped. Her social life had also become restricted since her divorce. The wasted lungs mirrored Nicole's belief that she was wasting her life—not only her physical life, but her inner life as well. Nicole described her mother as loving, though judgmental and controlling. Each time they spoke, her mother's comments and tone of voice reminded her that she was no longer a *somebody*.

Through the drawing exercise, Nicole realized she could make different choices, which would enhance her healing. She decided to release the limiting belief that she was a nobody. Rather than replacing it with a new belief, she decided she would stay in the "don't know" space and see what happened.

This exercise is particularly healing for those who insist "I can't draw" and "I'm a terrible artist." If you hear negative comments regarding your work, remember that's not you, it's a member of the Committee, intent on sabotaging your effort. Now spend a few minutes with what you've done. Notice how you feel as you look at your work. If there's anything that you find powerful, surprising, or interesting, take some time out and write about it in your journal. In the next chapter you will continue working with this image to Undo it.

## ASTHMA SYMPTOMS— WHAT ELSE ARE THEY TELLING YOU?

By now, you have begun to create a different relationship with asthma symptoms. Instead of just trying to get rid of the symptom, as in conventional Western medicine, you are learning how to Focus on the symptom's meaning and message. For, until we listen to the message of the symptom, it continues to repeat itself in one form or another. If you hold a belief that physical symptoms have no meaning besides your bodily discomfort, we suggest you suspend this way of thinking. Your Committee will be more than glad to hold onto it for you until you decide you want it back.

When you listen without analyzing or drawing conclusions, symptoms reveal themselves. A symptom may speak to you during an imagery exercise, while writing in your journal, in a dream, or as a spontaneous insight that seems to come out of nowhere. This next section describes how Focusing through breathing, singing, and a unique exercise called the Breathometer (pronounced like barometer or thermometer) can shift your relationship to your symptoms and empower you to live joyfully and breathe freely.

## BreathWorks: Singing, Breathing, and Healing
How often do you fully release your breath? When, if ever, do you sing out with joy and let go of sadness and pent-up emotions? How important is the relationship of letting go to breathing? And what can singing offer in the process of channeling both breath and emotion?

On a video produced by the Carl Stough Institute of Breathing Coordination,[13] Lauren Flanigan, an operatic soprano and an asthmatic, describes her symptoms as claustrophobic. Claustrophobia involves a fear of being closed in, confined in a narrow space. It is the phobic concomitant of an asthma symptom. In Flanigan's case, her claustrophobic symptoms mirrored the torment of her emotional confinement to grief. Even the music she chose involved sadness, grieving, and loss. Chinese medicine sees grief as an important sign of "internal cold," which affects both the lungs and the adrenal glands. Grief makes it harder for us to breathe—it's what we "hold" in our chest or gut.[14]

Carl Stough, a conductor and musician, turned his interest and knowledge of singing and breathing into a breathing therapy for people with lung conditions: Stough taught Flanigan to think and breathe differently. "Life begins and ends on the exhalation," Stough says. Though many of us may find this surprising, Stough is right. It's the exhalation that is the key to life's beginning, just as it is the exhalation that ends it. He teaches his clients to stop holding their breath, to cease "confining" it, and he tells them it's all in the letting go. This refocusing of thought and breath helps the bodily organs and systems (the lungs, the diaphragm, the nervous and hormonal systems) to release and expand in ways that cannot be experienced otherwise. Quite naturally, the voice becomes stronger and more resonant. Under Stough's guidance, Flanigan learned to Focus on fully releasing her breath; in doing this, she began releasing her attachment to grief as well. This gave Flanigan the space she needed to rise to a new level in her singing and in her life. Where before she sang of grief, she now sang of joy.

Where and when do *you* hold your breath, hold on to grief, refuse to let go? The Breathometer exercise gives you the chance to make some potent observations regarding these issues.

## The Breathometer

A barometer is a scientific instrument that measures atmospheric pressure. But we also use the term as an indicator of other kinds of fluctuations that are not necessarily scientific. For example, opinion polls serve as a barometer of public likes and dislikes, or the tone of someone's voice may act as a barometer of his or her mood. The Breathometer is an indicator, as well. But, instead of attending to atmospheric pressures related to weather conditions, it indicates another kind of pressure in the atmosphere—the kind generated by the people, places, and situations in your life that provoke breath holding and induce asthma symptoms. The Breathometer shows how the changes in the atmosphere of your mental and emotional life affect how you breathe—and beyond this, how they can trigger an asthma attack or prevent one from coming on.

The simple Focusing exercise that follows gives you the opportunity to become aware of those times when you are breath holding, which is the first step toward breaking this unhealthy and damaging habit. It's not only asthmatics who hold their breath. All of us refuse to let go of things, including anger, resentment, grief over losses, stories about the past, youth, beauty, material possessions of every kind, and one another. Naturally (or unnaturally), we attach our anxiety, depression, sadness, fear, anger, tension, excitement to our breath, and we hold it. We do this whether we expect good news or are afraid of hearing the worst, and we do it even while we're asleep.

Breathing fully, particularly remembering to exhale fully, is a rare function for children as well as adults. When we forget to do this, the air that remains in our lungs, like the thoughts and feelings we hold onto in our minds, becomes stale and toxic. While all of us suffer the results of this habit, people with asthma suffer the most.

## THE BREATHOMETER EXERCISE

*Intention:* To Focus on breath holding.

*Frequency:* Use once, then again at any time you choose to Focus on this habit.

1. *Notice* when you are holding your breath.
2. *Label it.* As soon as you notice this behavior, label it "breath holding."
3. *Stop.* Once you label it, stop and ask yourself the following questions:

   Where am I ?

   What am I doing (or what is happening)?

   Who am I with?

   What am I thinking?

   What am I feeling?
4. *Exhale.* When you have completed the process, release your breath.

Breath holding often involves holding oneself to perfectionist expectations—living up to the standards of the Committee, for whom you are never good enough, or at best only as good as your last success. We forget to be in the present moment. An action as simple as washing dishes can start it off. You notice that you are holding your breath. You label it: "breath holding." Then you stop and ask yourself the Breathometer questions:

Where am I ?
*I am in my kitchen.*
What am I doing (or what is happening)?
*I am washing dishes.*
Who am I with?
*I am by myself (with my kids, with my spouse, and so forth).*
What am I thinking?
*I'm running out of soap; the baby is crying; I have more important things to do.*
What am I feeling?
*I am tired; bored; annoyed; pressured. I want to be somewhere else.*

The process is equally valuable for tracking symptoms. Follow the same steps as before:

1. *Notice it* (the symptom).
2. *Label it* ("symptom").
3. *Stop* and ask the questions you asked for breath holding.
4. *Exhale* and release the symptom along with your breath.

Remember to write down your answers, and keep track of them. See how they change. Notice any patterns. And veto all judgments imposed on you by the Committee.

Some other important questions you can ask yourself regarding breath holding are:

- What am I afraid to let go of ?
- What am I holding back?

- What am I holding on to?
- What am I trying to hold together?

Many people associate difficulty in exhaling, whether as a habit or a symptom, with holding back (or holding in) feelings. By doing this exercise to identify the feelings you experience during an asthma attack, or while holding your breath, you now have the chance to separate from them and even to release them.

## FOCUSING ON RELATIONSHIPS

At the core of all healing lies the issue of relationship: the relationship of body and mind, of organs and systems, of the invisible world to the visible, of person to person, and of each individual to a Higher Power or to God. From the mindbody perspective, all illness is sociorelational, not isolated or random. Thus, in the final part of this chapter, we Focus on the relationships we live out in our daily lives with all this entails—from the heights of joyfulness to the depths of despair.

Relationship begins with your birth family and spirals outward to include friendship, love, parenting, work, and spiritual development. When you Focus on asthma as sociorelational, you might ask yourself *who* you are allergic to, as well as what. For example: Is it the feather filling in your mother's (sister's, friend's) down sofa that makes you wheeze? Or is it your relationship with the person, or persons, who live there and what this embodies? In all likelihood, it's both. This doesn't imply that you should blame someone else for your problem. Whether it be asthma or any other difficulty, once you recognize the importance of relationship in healing (and in healing relationships) you may begin to consider this disease from a more integrated stance—one that encourages you to look at the bigger picture. When you begin to watch, to listen, and to be in the present moment, you may discover uncharted territory that you can now claim for your own.

## Suffocated by Love

Melanie is an asthmatic who has been in a difficult, unsatisfying marriage for sixteen years. From the day she married Alan, she felt like she couldn't breathe. Melanie knew the relationship was stifling and that it would benefit her health to leave, and she had been on the verge of doing this many times in the past. But Melanie was torn apart by two opposing wishes—one to stay, thus ensuring familiarity no matter how painful the status quo, the other to go, which involved unseating herself and risking the unknown.

When Melanie's asthma surfaced in acute form, it was the knock at the door that she had been dreading. Her dilemma had begun long before when her Committee convinced her that life was supposed to be a certain way—that she needed the security and prestige of being married; that her children had to attend the right schools and live in the best neighborhood; and that she was ill prepared to face life on her own. Melanie had made up a story about the future and was intent on living it out no matter what. She hated staying, and she was afraid of leaving. So she remained stuck in a situation that took her breath away.[15] By resisting the truth, she became the slave of the Committee. And by refusing to risk the discomfort of being in the "don't know" space, she forfeited both her freedom and health.

Melanie's error is shared by many of us who confuse aloneness with loneliness, and separateness with isolation: we fall into the hole as described by the poem we looked at in the previous chapter. We are attached to the Committee's view of how life should be; we fear loss, deny the truth, refuse to take responsibility, and resist the changes that allow us to attain freedom. Being in relationship begins by Focusing on the relationship you have with *yourself*. It's not narcissism but necessity to look in the mirror and say (or at least think), "I *like* being me." There is life beyond the addictive, pop psychology of the "inner child" that complains about what it didn't get and blames parents for the ways they "failed" us. By acknowledging the need to release the past and by Focusing on who you are as an adult, you move toward forgiveness and acceptance of yourself and others, right here, right now. In our practice of this work we are fond of the saying: "I'm not okay. You're not okay. And that's okay." It's right up there with "I don't know." You see, if we don't need to be okay all the time, and we don't weigh ourselves down with having to know the answers, it's a lot easier to breathe.

## RELATIONSHIP AS A HEALING PRACTICE

Relationship is a healing practice. Our being together may have a far deeper meaning than we realize. It brings our character flaws and unresolved issues clearly into focus and encourages us to perfect ourselves. Our interactions with others, especially others with whom we are close, act as a magnifying glass and a magnet for the beliefs, feelings, thoughts, and behaviors we attach to so closely they become invisible. If we "bend over backward," "walk on eggshells," or "refuse to rock the boat," we compromise ourselves and prevent true communion. This keeps us, as well as the other person, stuck, and it precludes any sense of separation or detachment. Therefore, if I am not separate from you and you are not separate from me, neither of us has room to breathe. It is not coincidental that we use the words "You take my breath away" when we are overwhelmed with deep feelings for another person.

Being in a loving relationship is a gift as well as a practice. It is about more than the obvious issues of romance, attraction, comfort, and security. Loving relationships allow you to experience life in a way that may not always be without pain yet can offer the opportunity to polish the gemstone of your nature. When asthma symptoms arise, whether they manifest as your own or a family member's, they provide opportunities to make the necessary healing changes.

The following imagery exercise is one that gives you a chance to Focus on and nurture your primary relationship—the one with yourself, which so deeply affects the ones you have with others. If you choose, you may use this exercise to begin the day for the next 21 days.

---

### TWO OF YOU [16]

Close your eyes and breathe out three times.

Imagine there are two of you and that one of you is sitting on your lap.

And that you are hugging yourself.

And that you are holding your own face in your hands.

What happens? How do you feel? Then breathe out and open your eyes.

---

Some people find it difficult to hug themselves in adult form. They reduce themselves to child size. They use images of their children, grandchildren, nieces, and nephews instead. If it's this difficult to love ourselves in our imagination, where anything is possible, it makes sense that it would be even more difficult in our everyday lives. Since joy is the primary mind medicine to open and heal the lungs, and love is so deeply related to joy, it's not hard to see the importance of making a correction. You might ask yourself: What beliefs do I have that prevent me from loving myself as I am? Do I deserve affection? Am I worth it?

The first time Nick, a sixty-five-year-old retiree with acute asthmatic symptoms, tried to imagine he was hugging himself, he found it impossible. Instead, he hugged his grandson. Later, he realized he had skipped a generation by passing over his son; even that felt too close. At the end of 21 days, however, the process of imagery had worked its magic; Nick was able to imaginally hold his face in his hands quite tenderly. He explained how doing this gave him a feeling of warmth that he had missed as a child and had feared as an adult. When Nick stayed with his discomfort, not complaining or judging it, it became an act of healing. If you feel as Nick did, that hugging yourself is awkward and uncomfortable, the key is not to run away but to turn toward the discomfort and embrace it. You can do this by continuing to practice this exercise. Whatever disturbance you experience is a signal that treating yourself in a loving way is just the kind of mind medicine you need.

In this chapter you have learned the importance of the Focusing process, which is the foundation of FUN. By paying attention in this new way, you've seen how beliefs, symptoms, and relationships mirror one another in an ongoing body-mind dance. Now that you can see and hear the message of your difficulties more clearly, you can start undoing them. The Undoing process is the next step of the FUN program, which you will read about in the following chapter. Before going on, however, review the Focusing Essentials to remind yourself of what you have just learned:

*The Essentials of Focusing*
1. *Become the Watcher.* Use this concept to concentrate without effort, to observe without judging, no matter what the difficulty.
2. *Dismember the Committee.* Know these false selves for who they are. Recognize and release them.
3. *Defuse the dangers of nocebos.* Identify the negative beliefs about your health that are carelessly planted as truths. Then separate from them.
4. *Listen to your symptoms* without judging them. Acknowledge what they tell you.
5. *Make a separation* from your beliefs, symptoms, and relationships, and create the space of freedom.
6. *Take responsibility.* Asthma is sociorelational. Watch how you feel with the various people in your life, without blaming them for the asthma.
7. *Focus on joy.* It's joy that heals the lungs.

### CHAPTER 7

# UNDO

## *Create the Healing Turn*

*You have power you never dreamed of. . . . There are no
limitations to what you can do except the limitations of
your own mind.*

DARWIN P. KINGSLEY

---

**UNDO**

- Old George/New George
- Undo with Opposites
- The Ultimate Undoer
- Writing to Heal
- Using the Shocks
- Dream Medicine
- Your Own Top 20

---

In this chapter you take what you gained through Focusing and learn to Undo, the next part of FUN. As we mentioned in the introduction, Undoing is comparable to using the undo icon on your computer screen; what you have done is undone without discussion, guilt, or blame. Of course, Undoing goes much deeper than that, especially when you use the technique of imagery and enter the invisible world of imagination. Here, what you may have thought could never be Undone becomes a whole different story (or image)—one you can deal with in a way that even modern science has begun to recognize as powerful and healing.

Learning to Undo is a great challenge. When we are faced with issues and symptoms that we have dealt with for years, our habit is to recoil, to insist these things can't be changed. But remember, that's the Committee talking. The following anecdote shows how one of the most Committee-driven characters in our popular culture stumbled onto the technique of Undoing and used it to turn his life around. Along with many healing exercises, including some powerful imagery, a newly researched technique in writing, and an enjoyable way to integrate music into your healing plan, this chapter holds many valuable surprises. First, George's story.

## OLD GEORGE, NEW GEORGE

After a nine-year run, the TV comedy *Seinfeld* departed the airwaves, taking with it George Costanza, one of the least lovable television characters of all time. George was the ultimate loser. With an abrasive personality, a pessimistic outlook, and a talent for losing jobs and for striking out with women, he sought approval in ways guaranteed to ensure failure. Even his Committee couldn't make him more miserable than he made himself. But on one particular episode, George took a flyer that turned things around. Suddenly he became a new person—a confident, devil-may-care, magnetic winner.

The key to George's success was that in any situation—with women, work, food, friends—no matter what he would have done in the past, he now did the opposite. Where the old George would be shy, the new George acted bold; where the old George would make excuses, the new George quickly admitted his errors; where the old George would hide in the background, the new George dared to step forward. He had become what he had never dared imagine, his own hero, "Opposite Man."

By breaking his habits of telling stories and making judgments, George unwittingly managed to Undo. In that instant he walked through the mirror to the other side and leaped into a new life. Since his intention was not to grow and heal but rather to deliver a half hour of amusement to millions of viewers, by the following week he was back to his old self, exactly where the producers needed him to be.

George didn't realize that as Opposite Man he had tapped into his limiting beliefs about what he could be, do, and accomplish and had spontaneously Undone them. What had been impossible for him all his life was suddenly a reality, and he was overcome with joy. Yet, since George's experience had been achieved without focus, intention, or awareness, his Committee easily regained its ground, and by the next episode he was back to "normal."

Does this sound at all familiar? Have you ever stepped out of character and experienced a surprising turn in your life? Somehow, you separate from your habits, allow things to happen differently, and they do! The Committee is caught asleep on the job, the false selves retire, at least temporarily, from the arena. The fear, the holding back, the habitual beliefs and stories about why this can't, won't, will never change vanish, and as if by magic transformation occurs. In this moment of Undoing, the old restraints and resistance unravel. And suddenly, you are *free!* Your *beliefs shift;* this is the key. The beliefs about who you are, what you deserve, what is possible, and what is not: it's your belief system that is the source, the nucleus, your mental DNA. George made the shift unwittingly. He hadn't a clue. But here, as part of FUN, you can use the principle of opposites to create your own transformation through the conscious use of intention and will.


## USING OPPOSITES TO UNDO AND HEAL

Using opposites and opposition to Undo our errors and create balance has been part of healing traditions for thousands of years. Although the Western mind thinks of opposition only in terms of difficulty, the I Ching, an ancient Chinese spiritual text, views the principle of opposites differently—with an eye toward the care and development of the soul. It tells us:

> In general, opposition appears as an obstruction ... but it also has its *useful and important function.* The oppositions of heaven and earth, spirit and nature, man and woman, when reconciled, bring about the creation and reproduction of life. In the world of visible things, the principle of opposites makes possible the *differentiation* ... through which order is brought into the world.[1]

It's clear that without opposites and opposition there would be no chance for defining ourselves as individuals and for enlivening our relationships. If all things were similar or the same, to whom, or what, would we relate? Thus, what is often looked at as bad, like a symptom or difficulty, once again can turn out to be just the opposite. By making us feel uncomfortable, the opposites, differences, and difficulties in life provide us with a knock at the door. When we listen to them they can serve us as wake-up calls that keep our energy flowing instead of allowing it to stagnate.

In the previous chapter, we listed ten beliefs about asthma that your Committee thrives on. These beliefs rely heavily on judgments, standards, complaining, blaming, shaming, comparing, and telling threatening stories about the future. If you think you are not caught up in this kind of thinking, listen to how often you use the words *should, ought,* or *must,* and observe how concerned you are about being normal, perfect, accepted, approved of, and important. At one time or another, all of us fall into this trap, especially when it relates to an illness or difficulty that's chronic, another favorite word of both the Committee and conventional medicine. The question is, how do we Undo this habitual self-victimizing pattern?

The following exercise, called "Turning Things Around," expands upon what you learned in chapter 3 in the "Exercise for

Panic Prevention." It gives you a chance to use what you have learned about Focusing to generate the act of Undoing. This is how you begin. As soon as you catch yourself thinking or saying anything limiting, negative, or that hints of the Committee's agenda (such as the beliefs about asthma we just mentioned) you write it down. Next, you immediately think of a thought or belief to reverse this, one that may be its opposite. You write this down as well, no matter how ridiculous, impossible, or naive it may seem. Remember that this mental static (*ridiculous, impossible, naive*) is the Committee squawking, balking, and talking, becoming even more desperate for control as you take steps to Undo the damage it has so diligently spent your entire life masterminding.

This exercise is one of the most practical and powerful ways to begin Undoing your enslavement to the Committee. The expression *to turn things around* is a familiar one that involves a turn of mind and a change of heart. In making this kind of turn you move to the high ground—a place the Committee dares not go for fear of being Undone themselves when exposed by the light of freedom and truth.

---

## TURNING THINGS AROUND

*Intention:* To confront and disempower the Committee. To transform the feelings, thoughts, words, and beliefs that pull you down and keep you stuck. These may include any nocebos (the bad seed-thoughts) planted by authority figures, the media, family, friends, and statistics.

*Frequency:* To be done every time you notice yourself saying or thinking any of the above.

Whenever you notice yourself thinking or saying anything limiting or that smacks of negativity—stop!

Take out your notebook or journal (you might want to keep a

---

special, pocket-sized one for this purpose) and write down this thought or feeling.

Do not judge, censor, or analyze what you write.

Now, without thinking about it, write the opposite thought—one that reverses or can Undo the first, that turns it around. Keep this thought in the present. If your worry or concern is about the future, remind yourself that the future is something we make up, a story that doesn't exist.

For instance, your thought might be "I'm feeling tied down." Or "I will never be free of this illness." Once you have written it down, the thought or belief is made visible. It's out in the open. This has the same effect as the water that's thrown on the Wicked Witch of the West in *The Wizard of Oz*. She begins to melt, and even her henchmen rejoice. When you consciously expose your thoughts instead of telling stories about what might happen in the future or complaining, it's much the same. Suddenly, you are no longer enslaved, and you are set free to think and do the opposite. In this case the opposite might be (for either or both of these), "I am free as a bird"—or whatever you naturally come up with. You may also convert some of these thoughts into images. The one we just did would be simple. You simply close your eyes, breathe out three times, and:

- See yourself *tied down*.
- Then you breathe out again, and see yourself *free as a bird*.

Do this now and see what happens. Another example might be "I feel blue." To make this into an image, you would see yourself feeling blue. Then you imagine the opposite. One client actually saw that she had turned blue. When she imagined the opposite, she spontaneously saw herself turn a glowing pink. She immediately felt happier, healthier, "in the pink."

Choose three to five thoughts to practice with. They don't have to be about asthma. They can be anything that the Committee sends your way. If you do this consistently, you soon will be able to identify your recurring thought patterns and Undo them. If you find yourself rebelling against this exercise, not wanting to bother to write things down, and doubting that something so simple can produce results, guess who's talking! We suggest that you practice this exercise for at least a week and see what happens before you allow the Judge to veto it or the Skeptic to sow the seeds of doubt.

By practicing these acts of self-remembering, you restore yourself to life.[2] Think of them as imaginal habit breakers that for an instant allow you to leave behind your difficulty and take a leap into freedom. Don't worry about whether your choice of an opposite is far-fetched or impossible. In the world of imagination, *anything* is possible. And once you get a taste of making the impossible become possible *there*, you can change your belief and do it *here* as well. Even when asthma isn't directly mentioned, its underlying mental, emotional, social, and moral issues are all addressed—grief, anger, perfectionism, power, isolation, self-worth, enslavement, freedom, love, loss, and truth.


## IMAGINATION: THE ULTIMATE UNDOER

Imagery is a powerful mind technology for Undoing. The exercises in this chapter are effective for Undoing beliefs, for removing symptoms, and for healing relationships. They help you live an asthma-free life. The next story reveals how closely the heart and the lungs are linked.

### Getting to the Heart of Things: A Journey via Imagination

Dr. Martin Rossman had been using imagery successfully with a twenty-four-year-old man with a long history of asthma when suddenly the asthma symptoms returned. Dr. Rossman suggested to his client that he imagine going inside his chest to see what was going on. Once inside, the client reported there was an agitated dwarf guarding the territory leading to his heart. When anyone came too close, the dwarf blocked the entrance, which initially appeared as a tunnel. Not coincidentally, the tunnel looked like a bronchial tube, which closed down when the dwarf sounded the warning of a possible invasion.[3]

Instead of an intellectual insight, this imagery provides a lived experience of the difficulty. The recurrence of the physical symptoms is related to the habit of closing down emotionally whenever this man becomes involved in a romantic relationship. The dwarf mirrors his stunted emotional growth as well as his mistrust and isolation. The connection between feelings and asthma is a strong one. Though love is a powerful healer, because of certain beliefs, many of us resist it. We fear the pain it may cause, the weakness it reveals, or the difficult issues it brings up. For asthmatics, the fears of suffocation, of being held too close, of not being held at all, and of separation and loss are enough to cause breathing problems.

The image of the dwarf guarding the way to the heart, which also turns out to be a tunnel leading to the lungs, reveals how entwined the heart and the lungs really are. When your imagery brings you face-to-face with a truth such as this, it's impossible to rationalize or ignore it. This experience alone creates an immediate shift in awareness. Since imagination is unlimited, there are many ways to Undo the self-protective beliefs that create this limiting circumstance.

How would you take care of this difficulty? Would you banish the dwarf? Befriend him? *Become* him? If one image doesn't work, try another. An appropriate and effective way of Undoing the dwarf might involve doing the *opposite* of what you would do ordinarily. If you tend to fear confrontation and your habit is to try and slip past, you might have a go with the dwarf head-on. You will know if your imagery is on target by the way you feel and how your body responds.

## IMAGERY FOR UNDOING

The imagery exercises that follow are specifically geared toward Undoing the condition of asthma. This includes eliminating, reversing, and releasing the beliefs, symptoms, and circumstances that create, exacerbate, and maintain it. You can do those that appeal to you as you read along, or you can use the ones that interest you once you have finished the chapter.

"The Exorcism" provides a healing for the lungs that addresses the physical symptoms yet goes far deeper. Issues of freedom, relationship, and truth are also strongly involved. Thus we refer to it as laying the groundwork for true recovery. It eliminates the symptom by going to the root—getting whoever or whatever is interfering with your breathing to reveal itself. Because it is long, you may want to put it on tape, read it over a couple of times before doing it, or have someone read it to you. Don't be concerned if this exercise stirs up feelings of guilt or pain. No matter what your Committee says, this exercise will not cause you or anyone else harm.

---

### THE EXORCISM [4] *

*Intention:* To heal the lungs.

*Frequency:* Use it in the morning for up to three minutes (for one minute anytime you experience wheezing) for seven days.

Close your eyes and breathe out three times. See yourself taking off your clothes. See yourself in a mirror nude from the neck down. In the mirror, with your right forefinger (the left if you are left-handed) touch on or into your upper chest area from the front all the way around to the back, making a complete circle. Now touch the area of greatest discomfort, and see who isn't allowing you to breathe, that is, see whose face appears in the area. Who is restricting your breathing, and what color appears there? Breathe out that

---

color in long, slow exhalations while removing from the area whomever you've seen, at first as gently as you can. If the person does not leave easily, use increasing force, going from the gentle to the vigorous, perhaps eventually going so far as to use a golden scalpel to cut the person out. As you are removing this person, tell him or her that he or she is no longer permitted to stay in your body, that he or she has to leave and stay a far distance from your body; that he or she is no longer welcome in your body and will never be allowed to enter your body again. After the removal, see yourself becoming very, very tall and reaching your arms far up into the sky, all the way to the sun. Take a piece of the sun in your palms and place it in the vacated space. See the area healing, and see how you look and feel. Then, put your clothes back on, breathe out once, and open your eyes, knowing that you are breathing easily.

This exercise reveals the difficulty many of us have in telling the difference between dependency and love. It's not surprising that those we are closest to appear and that removing them from our lungs may be painful. Acknowledging how enmeshed your breathing is with close relationships may bring up feelings of sadness, loss, resentment, or even guilt, but it is important not to label these feelings as bad or to bury them. Actually, the opposite is true. For, as you'll see in the next story, it's only when we recognize these feelings and bring them into the open that we create the necessary space to heal.

## Bamboozled by the Committee

Karen, a business executive in her late thirties, had her first asthma attack when she was seventeen. For the last eight years she has lived with Michael, with whom she shares parenting responsibilities for his five-year-old son. When she does "The Exorcism," Karen sees her mother and cuts her out. She gets a sense of power from this. When she's finished she says her breathing seems much easier. But Karen is disturbed by the feeling of guilt that washes over her almost immediately. She describes her mother as a worrier and overprotective. "She's afraid I can't take care of myself. She's a typical Jewish mother," Karen adds with exasperation.

Karen did the exercise for less than a week. She claimed it made her feel guilty. "I've discussed this stuff with my therapist for the past six years. Why do it again?" she asked. Talking with her therapist about her mother was a safe way for Karen to dwell on her pain. It allowed her to vent (complain, name, blame, be the victim), but it made no impact on the asthma. Despite feeling powerful and breathing more freely after her initial imagery experience, Karen allowed her Committee to take over. The Judge pronounced her guilty, based on standards that dictate a "good" daughter's behavior. And immediately, Karen fell into the trap of thinking that removing her mother's image and influence from her lungs was "bad."

Regarding the emotional issues of asthma and their relationship to its symptoms, Dr. Gerald Epstein says:

> The emotional contribution (of asthma) seems to come mainly from knotted dependency problems, particularly related to struggles for independence from maternal influence, although sometimes the distressing influence can be paternal. Either way . . . the issue is almost always related to a parent. The asthmatic wheeze has a positive as well as a negative meaning. The positive meaning is expression of wanting to breathe freely—to become free. The negative meaning is generally considered to bespeak the fear of breaking loose from parental influence.[5]

The more resistance you have to this idea, the more likely it is to have personal value. Whether or not you believe it is true, don't replicate Karen's error. Karen tears herself apart through living out this asthmatic double bind. On the one hand she is disdainful of her "typical" Jewish mother (the worrier) and seeks freedom from her dominance, while on the other she becomes paralyzed by guilt when she tries to remove her. The symptoms of asthma mirror her two opposing wishes—to become independent and free and to remain dependent and enslaved—and are quick to follow. So are the two inhalers she uses to control her wheezing. The bottom line is clear: Karen is bamboozled by her Committee. She prefers complaining to her therapist and treating the symptoms of the asthma to taking a risk that might cause some initial pain but eventually set her free.

When you do this exercise yourself, whether the person (or persons) you find inside go easily or need to be extracted with a golden scalpel, the Committee may try to meddle, as it did with Karen. It may send in the Victimizer to plant seeds of guilt with the intention of deterring you from getting unstuck, both from the person who is interfering with your breathing and from the asthma. If this happens, stop and do this next exercise. If not, proceed to "Less Is More."

## CASTING OUT THE VICTIMIZER

*Intention:* To Undo any member(s) of the Committee.

*Frequency:* To be used whenever needed, for up to one minute, the first time. Then for thirty seconds. Then fifteen seconds. Since imagery occurs outside linear time, as you become accustomed to the process you can move through it more quickly without sacrificing its effect. In fact, by doing it without dwelling, the Committee member being cast out gets the message even more clearly. It's like throwing a switch. Flick, and it's done.

Close your eyes and breathe out three times. See the Victimizer (or any other Committee member who appears) inside you. Once you have seen this, breathe out again. Now cast this intruder out of your body (much the same way you just used in "The Exorcism").

Bring along anything you might need to help you—a scalpel, a
rope, even a hook, like they once used in vaudeville to haul a loser
off stage. Tell the intruder it must leave and not return. Once it
departs, breathe out and open your eyes.

## Less Is More

Since all Committee members are fully vested in retaining the
status quo, they try to return. But from now on this technique for
getting rid of them is at your disposal. The more quickly you do
this exercise, the less chance they have to draw you toward the
familiar hole that they have so skillfully dug for you.

Carol, a forty-eight-year-old asthmatic, had been knuckling
under to her Committee members for years. She finally got fed up
with their antics and decided to Undo them. After a demeaning
conversation with a co-worker, Carol was about to forsake a
research project she had collaborated on for eighteen months.
Closing her eyes, she found not one Committee member but a
coven of them, dancing around a steaming cauldron and cackling
about how they had won again. In an instant she saw how her failure to attain completion was her own creation, born of her pattern
of perfectionism and feelings of guilt. By dousing the Committee
with water, she put a damper on their celebration, cooled the
flames of her anger, and regained her perspective. This allowed her
the space to successfully complete the project without worrying
about living up to the Committee's impossibly high standards.

## HEALING THE PAST

Our choice of imagery reflects who we are. What one of us finds
disquieting, another may find liberating. When Amy did "The
Exorcism," she was quick to remove her mother, along with sev-

eral others who appeared, working on each person for seven days or until he or she was completely gone from her body. Amy said her mother had never really been there for her except at her convenience or when she felt needy. Then Mom would pull her close, restricting her life with her needs and demands, only to abandon her once again when her needs changed or were met by someone else. Using the exercise made Amy feel more open. Within a couple of weeks the number of asthma attacks was cut in half. After relieving her symptoms with "The Exorcism," Amy felt ready to confront a memory of sexual abuse from the time she was six. Though she could not actually change what had happened back then, she was able to change her attitude, memory, and response toward it by using the next imagery exercise, "Hands of Time."

---

### HANDS OF TIME[6]

*Intention:* To Undo a distressing or traumatic event of the past.

*Frequency:* Every morning for seven days, for no longer than two minutes.

Close your eyes and breathe out three times. See before you a clock. Imagine where the hands of the clock are now (at the moment you are doing this exercise). Now breathe out one time slowly and turn the hands back to the inner or outer event in your past that distresses you. See this event happening now, as it did then. . . . Breathe out one time, and imagine yourself doing something to correct this experience. Remember that anything is possible in the imagination. When you are finished, turn the hands of the clock forward to the present time. Sense, know, and live how your emotions and physiology have harmonized.

---

We are "less damaged by the traumas of childhood, than by the traumatic way we *remember* childhood."[7] Remembering and rehashing past events keeps us enslaved, justifying our pain by forever insisting we were victims. But through using imagination we have a chance to do more. Since what we can do, see, or be in imagination has no limits, Amy used this imagery exercise and returned to the scene of the abuse in a new way. With the strength she had gained from her previous imagery experience, she found herself able to Undo the past by simply walking away from this person. She saw herself getting up, opening the door, leaving the room, and closing the door behind her. Immediately, her perception of the past, including her feelings and beliefs about it, shifted.

Any discussion of past events is irrelevant: people spend much of their time thinking, discussing, or denying, only to remain trapped. The experience that had haunted Amy all her life was put to rest, first by transforming it, then by "closing the door" on it. From that time on, if any memories were triggered, she had the imagery to use as a buffer and a transformer.

Amy had gone from victim to victor in less than three minutes. She felt liberated and reborn. What she had accomplished was an Undoing of her perception of this past event. Amy had been living this event over and over again in her memory and was constantly open to reminders of it in her daily life. By using the exercise "Hands of Time," you too can Undo any burdensome memories that weigh you down and prevent you from moving forward.

## RECENT RESEARCH: WRITING HEALS ASTHMA

Has the Doubter put in an appearance yet, claiming that Undoing the past can't possibly relieve asthma symptoms? Has he insisted that you be logical, use good common sense, and look at this from a scientific point of view? Wonderful! According to a recent study on the effects that writing about stressful experiences has on the symptoms of asthma, he hasn't a leg to stand on. This study used writing instead of imagery, yet the results are similar—including the statistics. Researchers asked patients to draw on their inner beliefs, thoughts, and feelings about a past event and to experience them within a creative context. According to this controlled clinical trial, thirty-nine asthma patients completed an experiment in which they wrote about the most stressful event of their lives. They did this for twenty minutes on three consecutive days a week for one week and were evaluated at two weeks, two months, and four months after treatment. Starting at two weeks, 47 percent of the patients who were treated showed clinically relevant changes in lung function, as compared with changes of 24 percent in the control group.[8]

This rigorous study, conducted at the State University of New York, Stony Brook, School of Medicine by Dr. Joshua M. Smyth, is the first to prove that writing about stressful life experiences improves physician ratings of disease severity and objective physiological markers. While participating patients wrote about their most stressful experience, control group patients wrote about their daily activities. All were asked to write continuously, without regard for spelling, style, or other artistic or editorial concerns, and were signaled to stop after twenty minutes. They could write about one topic for three sessions or could move from one topic to another. None of the work was discussed with staff or with other participants in the study. Most often, they wrote about deaths of loved ones, serious relationship problems, disturbing events of childhood, or occasionally of seeing or being involved in a major disaster.

Those who decide to use this technique must be willing to go the course: this means to write for the full twenty minutes, for three days, about something that matters, something really distressing, not just the events of the day. As Dr. Smyth observed, and as the Awfulizer will surely point out, this can be painful. Yet its value is enormous. By writing about the stress or trauma, you bring to the surface emotions and memories that may have been stuck inside you for years, and you expel them. This of itself is a kind of exorcism. If you choose to do this, follow these simple directions:

# WRITING TO HEAL

*Intention:* To heal the symptoms of the disease.

*Frequency:* Write for twenty minutes nonstop on three consecutive days.

Find a quiet place in which to write, and choose a stressful or traumatic past event or situation that you are willing to write about. We suggest that you handwrite this instead of using a computer, so the feelings flow through you and onto the paper.

Write for twenty minutes without stopping, and with no regard for how this looks or sounds or if it's correct or "good."

If feelings come up as you write, let them.

Do this for three days, always writing about a stressful event, even if it's not the same one. Do not discuss this process with others.

See what happens.

## UNDOING BY DRAWING

Drawing, like writing and imaging, has the power to Undo and to heal. In this case we advise that you go directly to the asthma and draw it. Whereas in chapter 6 you drew the asthma in order to Focus, now you draw the asthma with the intention of Undoing it. Drawing sets up lines of communication that bypass ordinary thinking and relate new messages to the body-mind.

In the "Decreating by Drawing" exercise you spend fifteen minutes drawing the asthma—whether that's the way you feel and look when you have an attack or a symptom or the symptom itself as an abstract shape or form. Then you find a way to contain, reverse, or eliminate it. This work is for your eyes only. Express yourself freely. Let go of your expectations of what this should look like. Intellectualizing and analyzing have no place in this process—they get between yourself and your drawing experience. This technique serves as a reminder to your body of what you want—to release, to reverse, to Undo the asthma. There's no need to be a "good" artist or to make an acceptable representation. The steps for decreating, which is a way of Undoing, through drawing are simple:

## DECREATING BY DRAWING

*Intention:* To reverse or Undo the asthma symptoms.

*Frequency:* Do once.

On a sheet of paper, draw and color the disease or the symptom. Let your imagination guide you, and allow the disease or symptom to reveal itself without the censorship of your Committee. What it looks like makes no difference.

After you complete this, on the same piece of paper Undo the image of the difficulty: destroy, eliminate, confine, or in any way you choose, transform it.

Keep this in a place where you will see it, and use it as a constant reminder of your intention to Undo the disease and render it harmless.

Traditional Western medicine has used this technique for centuries as a healing treatment. Equally valuable for children and adults, it is something anyone can do and have FUN with. One woman, whose disease appeared as a giant, dark weight on her chest, had a band of angels come and carry it away. As they lifted the weight, she immediately began to experience a sense of relief and release, both physically and emotionally. Another person drew his face as red and contorted during an attack. Then he drew himself smiling, laughing, and breathing freely. Both kept their drawings where they could easily see them. During the next few weeks they used them as reminders of the intention to break free of the debilitating symptoms of asthma.

Just as drawing can be valuable, another deeply healing element of natural medicine has always been dreams. If you want to become your own authority, one of the first places to look is the wisdom of your dreams. In this next section we introduce you to the dream process and lead you through an intriguing technique for Undoing those dreams that disturb you. Everything you have learned up till now is embedded in this one process—Focusing, belief work, imagery, art, writing, and an expanded sense of awareness. All this and more come together in a tapestry, uniquely your own, once you begin to work with your dreams.

## CREATING YOUR OWN DREAM MEDICINE

Dream life is the natural arena for dealing with the dynamics of life, inner and outer, and how they affect us. In the symbolic world of dreams we have a level of flexibility . . . lacking in the outer world. We have also in the inner life a greater potential for resolution. Whether in the inner or outer life *it is the lack of resolution which hangs us up.*[9]

Your dreams are wisdom that emerges from the clearest part of you—the part that sees, knows, and creates without limits. But most of us have never been taught the special language of dreams. We easily forget our dreams and rarely work with them; certainly, no medical doctor ever inquires about them. Dreams seem to compose a secret life to which few of us are privy. When we do show interest, the Committee is there in an instant to warn us away. Our dreams are the last thing it wants us to acknowledge as valuable. Of course, it's pointless to try to educate the Committee. It has no interest in learning that dreams have been used as an integral part of healing for thousands of years. It ignores the fact that some of the most renowned scholars and scientists, such as Descartes and Einstein, attributed their greatest discoveries to dreaming; that the ancient Greeks had special dream temples where people came to heal; or that this technique remains in use throughout the world. Yet, once you learn to listen to your dreams and to create your own personal dream medicine, the voices of the Committee will begin to seem weak in comparison.

## USING YOUR DREAMS

We've already described some of our clients' dreams and their relevance to the work. Linda's dream of the yellow-eyed wolf that turned into a man (chapter 5) and Bob's of the angry mob (chapter 6) are, like all dreams, mirrors. They reflect whatever is going on in your life; they tell you where you are now and of possibilities to come. They reveal what's happening with your health, in your relationships, in your work, and in the life of spirit. Dreams are not just random brain activity, the busy work of the sleeping mind. Becoming the Watcher of your dreams puts you in touch with wisdom that is ordinarily not available to you. Before going to sleep, you can ask yourself for dreams that will clarify the difficulties in relationships and the meaning and purpose of your symptoms. This leads to the discovery of previously secret knowledge that you can bring into waking life and integrate into your healing.

Once Linda understood that the yellow-eyed wolf was a part of herself rather than a frightening predator, she gained confidence and found inside herself a quality of power that had lain dormant. When Bob recognized that the angry mob reflected his own suppressed anger, he was able to own the anger and move past it. By making the effort to remember and write down your dreams, even the ones that seem most ridiculous, you gain access to that extraordinary part of yourself that refers you to your blueprint. Now, through the process of Undoing, you will learn to transform those dreams that are incomplete, frightening, or frustrating. With them, you may create your own personal dream medicine, a remedy that allows you to respond with courage instead of reacting out of fear.

## UNDOING AND RECONSTRUCTING YOUR DREAM

Have you ever had a dream where you have been pursued or felt threatened? What kind of feelings did it leave you with? Did you feel frightened, frustrated, victimized? Ordinarily we call these dreams nightmares and deliberately devalue and ignore them. But in doing this work, Bob realized this dream provided him with an opportunity to change his stance. He wanted to break free of the loop of enslavement he had created by choosing to act with courage instead of reacting out of fear. Undoing the dream made this possible.

### Reconstructing Bob's Dream

In the first part of the Undoing process, Bob recognizes the dream as a mirror of his own anger, which reveals itself in the form of the angry mob. Next he does the opposite of running away and instead confronts this mob. Bob uses a technique where he closes his eyes, and after a brief breathing process, described later in "Create Your Own Dream Medicine," he returns to the dream.[10] He sees himself running from the mob. At this point, Bob comes to the edge of a rooftop. Here he stops and confronts the mob with the awareness that in imagination and dreams all things are possible. He now uses his will and intention and makes a turn, both figuratively and literally, that brings him face-to-face with his pursuers. To respond in this way is an act of faith, an Undoing of his fear. As he looks the leader in the eyes, he watches the anger dissolve, and in its place is a deep sadness. The mob members become smaller, sinking down to the tar surface of the rooftop, and begin crying like children. At first Bob watches, then he embraces them. He feels as if something is cracking open inside himself in the region of his heart. As he does this, the anger vanishes. In its place is a feeling of acceptance—of the children and of their loss and grief. At the moment, this is enough. There is no need to fix it or to squelch the sadness as though it has no value.

## Valuing the Shocks

Bob feels cleansed and relieved. Initially, he had feared a battle where he would either slay or be slain. By embracing the weeping children in the dream he has embraced the sad-child quality of himself. He admits to being shocked by what happened. According to Madame Colette Aboulker-Muscat, a renowned teacher of imagery and dream work, it's just this shock that is necessary: it provokes a stress on the organism, which responds by trying to overcome the stress, thus generating movement and healing.

"We are transformed by our interaction with the environ-ment."[11] And not all these interactions need be pleasurable to be rewarding. Since often we are unconscious, or at least so deeply asleep that any movement in our lives is negligible, we need these shocks to make healing and rejuvenation possible. After the dream reconstruction, Bob writes and draws this experience in his note-book, giving it a title, dating it, and signing his name at the end. It's not important for him to analyze his experience, to find out who made him sad, or to understand what his sadness means. Though this kind of psychological insight is interesting, too often it becomes a trap. It's living out this experience in imagination that leads to his evolution and healing.

As Bob uses the exercise for the next 21 days, the process keeps changing. He has several different experiences along the way, both in his imagery and in his waking life. The children may cry or laugh; the night changes into day; the rooftop becomes a meadow, then leads him down to a river. And as he releases his long-held emotions of anger and sadness, he notices a change in his breathing as well. It becomes freer, less constricted, and the asthma attacks start to grow further and further apart. This one experience can't ensure that Bob will never feel angry or sad again; neither does it guarantee that his breathing will always be unrestricted. However, it does give him a technique that enables him to accept and inte-grate these feelings into his waking life. If you would like to create some similar dream medicine for yourself, here is the way to do it:

# CREATE YOUR OWN DREAM MEDICINE

*Intention:* To Undo a symptom or difficulty by *re-visioning* your dream.

*Frequency:* Do this exercise for the next 21 days, for up to three minutes each day.

Sit quietly, close your eyes, and count down silently from five to one, combining each number with an exhalation. When you reach one, breathe out, see the one become a zero, then see the zero grow larger and become a mirror.

Imagine that you are stepping through the mirror and returning to the dream.

Now go on with the dream in a new way. Undo your fear, anger, asthma, grief. Create new options and actions by bringing with you the knowledge that anything is possible in imagination. If it is dark, imagine bringing a light so you can see. If you need protection or anything to help you accomplish your task, imagine bringing these as well.

Once you have accomplished your task, notice how you feel, then return through the mirror, seeing yourself with a new attitude, feeling, and sense of yourself.

Before you exit the mirror, imagine pushing this image off with your right hand to the right, which indicates the future. (If you are left-handed, imagine pushing it off to the left.)

Count back up from one to five, with each new breath being a new number. Then open your eyes and return.

Write and draw what happens in your notebook. Date and sign your work.

# LIVING IN TUNE: UNDOING THROUGH
# THE POWER OF MUSIC

Just as dreams are legendary in their power to heal, so is music, which is the next and final part of the Undoing process. In the Old Testament and the I Ching, music was considered inspirational, sacred, and healing. The Greek philosopher Democritus wrote about the curative powers that emanate from the music of a simple flute. Indigenous cultures throughout the world have always used music to express the range of human emotion as well as mark rites and passages in a person's life. Today, music still flourishes. The forms are endless: jazz, rock, rap, rhythm and blues, show tunes, folk, classical, liturgical, orchestral, operatic, and so on.

In *The Mozart Effect*,[12] Don Campbell calls music the "common tongue" of the modern world and tells us it can replace costly medical treatments. This is not as far-fetched as it seems. Campbell's own experience with healing a blood clot in his brain is part of some convincing proof he brings to bear. It's nothing new to hear that "music hath charms that *soothe*...." It can also energize, excite, inflame, rejuvenate, and cleanse us; it inspires love, compassion, and faith. From Brahms's "Lullaby" to the Rolling Stones' "You Can't Always Get What You Want," music moves us in ways that words can never express. Talking about our disappointment, loneliness, or grief helps us vent, but it rarely gets us beyond our trouble, while the experience of listening to, playing, or creating music is genuinely therapeutic.

## MUSIC TO BREATHE BY

Long before music was used as entertainment, it was used as a source of healing. Like your dreams and imagery, music embodies feelings and beliefs; moods, hopes, fears, and possibilities. When music speaks to you through a specific lyric or sound, it becomes part of you and infuses you with its power to illuminate and heal.

## Create Your Own Top Twenty

Using music as a healing technique goes beyond just turning on the radio or slipping in your favorite CD and getting lost inside the sound pouring out of the speakers. When you listen to music as a reflection of where you are and what you are feeling in your life, it becomes an active, creative process. When you resonate with a particular piece, the next possibility is to tape it and to make it a part of your healing practice. To create your own top twenty, you may:

- Use pieces that you already know and love, that may already be a part of your music collection.
- Use music you find by listening to the radio or any other available source.
- Compose your own music and/or lyrics (or you may also compose lyrics for existing music).
- Listen to the tape you have made and make it a part of your life. Sing, dance, walk, run, cry, and laugh with it. Let it draw out your current feelings and open you up to new ones.

Once you make your healing tape, you will have created a musical hologram of your life. You can then go on to Undo those feelings that bring you down and make you feel "out of tune" or "out of sync." By changing the music, you change your mood and affect your beliefs and behavior. And the reverse is true as well: as your feelings and circumstances change, so will the music you choose to listen to. Remember Lauren Flanigan, who went from singing of grief to singing of joy? You too can do this. Consider replacing the music of despair with the music of joy, the music of heartbreak with the music of hope, the music of the places you have been with the music of places you have yet to go (even those unheard of in your wildest dreams).

This kind of listening is active listening, a technique cultivated with practice. To harmonize and balance the energies within yourself, allow the music to naturally enter your mind and heart. Use the music as mind medicine, just as you have used your imagery and dreams. You can also sing along, dance, run, and have FUN with it. Play your tape when you get up in the morning, again before you go to sleep at night, and anytime in between. Imagine every molecule of your body surrounded and filled to the brim with it. Change it whenever you want. Add new pieces. Undo or delete what no longer feels right. If you are more auditory than visual, this may be the perfect medicine for you. Use it however you wish to create your own unique healing prescriptions.

To complete this chapter, we would like to share a technique that you can use whenever your breathing feels constricted, or as a preventive prescription. Do it with eyes open or closed, according to your preference and the situation. This exercise, called the "Singing Lung," is particularly effective for those with exercise-induced asthma, which we will discuss in chapter 11. Use it while running or even while warming up. Know that by doing this you open your lungs and fill them with a healing balm created out of your own cornucopia of melodies, harmonies, lyrics, and rhythms.

## THE SINGING LUNG ❋

*Intention:* To Undo or prevent breathing difficulty. To have FUN!

*Frequency:* As often as you like.

This may be done with your eyes open or closed.

The next time your breathing gives you trouble, listen to a piece of music that relaxes, inspires, or energizes you. As you listen, begin to inhale the music—drawing it into your nose, down the back of your throat, and into your bronchial tubes. See and sense the bronchial tubes expanding and your lungs filling with white

light. Imagine your lungs smiling, happy, and singing along. See
and feel them expanding and become more and more radiant and
resilient. Continue until the end of the piece. Know you can use
this exercise at any time, with your tape or without. If you happen
to hear a piece of music that moves you as you're driving home
from work or while you're out walking or jogging, be spontaneous
and join in.

When you are done, breathe out, and if your eyes are closed,
open them and return.

## THE ESSENTIALS OF UNDOING

This is the point in the program where the challenge is greatest. It
is now that the members of your Committee are most likely to
warn you of danger and insist you should go back. The question
you might ask yourself here is, "Back to what?" To the asthma as it
was? To conventional medication as the only viable option? To a
belief system mired in stories of the past and enslaved to myths
about the future? We suggest that you tell the Committee, "Enough
is enough!" You have heard their song before, and it obviously
hasn't changed. Think, instead, of all you have already read and
accomplished and how much there is to gain. Remind yourself of
your intention in doing this work: look at your answers to part 4 of
the mindbody questionnaire in chapter 3, where you described how
it would be to live your life completely healthy and asthma free.
Decide what that's worth to you.

It's difficult enough to change your backhand in tennis, to start
a new job, or just to negotiate a parallel parking space. Here you
are being asked to Undo the way you think. Such a turn of mind is
not for the faint of heart. When Marilyn, a thirty-three-year-old
mother of twin girls, reached this point in the program, she likened

it to giving birth—specifically to that moment during labor when she decided it was time to go home. "This was more than I had bargained for," she said. "It was too much pain, too scary. I wanted to stop. Then *maybe* I would come back and try again when I felt rested and more in the mood. Getting to this place in the work felt the same," she said. "It was like giving birth all over again—not to a baby, but to a new way of living life. And I had no idea of how it would turn out or if I could really do it."

The stress Marilyn felt and that you may be feeling now is not the stress that we associate with exhaustion, helplessness, hopelessness, depressed immunity, and disease. It is, in fact, something known as "eustress" or good stress—stress that's beneficial, that strengthens your immune system and physiology. By choosing not to retreat and to go on to Now Act, you get the chance to put into action much of what you have already learned. We shape and heal ourselves—our minds, our souls, our spirit—by taking action in the everyday world. Mere contemplation won't do it for us. Through suggestions, exercises, and examples, chapter 8 provides the tools and opportunity to make that leap and to create a transformation in your health and in all areas of your life.

## The Essentials of Undoing

1. *Play with opposites.* Reverse what you ordinarily think and do. Even if it feels uncomfortable, think, say, and do the opposite. If you habitually defer, take over; if you usually fault yourself, give yourself credit; if you are quiet as a mouse, roar like a lion.
2. *Turn toward your difficulty.* Undo your impulse to label events, feelings, symptoms, and so forth as "bad." See what comes up for you as a challenge or opportunity instead of as a problem, and embrace it.
3. *Value the shocks.* Stop complaining about them. They can actually make you stronger and help you to grow.

4. *Heal the past* through the processes of imagery, writing, and dream work. Releasing grief, sadness, resentment, and anger makes room for joy. It's good mind medicine for the lungs.
5. *Live in tune.* Use the power of music to attune yourself to life, to generate joy, and to support your body's natural healing power.

### CHAPTER 8

# NOW ACT

## Heal by Having Fun

*Leap and the net will appear.*

JULIE CAMERON

**NOW ACT**

- Know by Doing
- Read the Glyphs
- Use Humor
- Create a Prayer Collage
- Seven Simple Action Generators
- Do unto Others
- Do unto Yourself

Focusing and Undoing—the *F* and *U* of FUN—have led you here. But now that you have arrived, what next? How do you take what you have learned and use it to generate action, fun, and healing in everyday life? The way is simple; you need look no further. You turn toward the asthma and acknowledge it as a catalyst—one that tells you it's time to change. And change occurs, not by gaining insight, watching television, or surfing the Internet, but through *taking action*. The next step is to Now Act.

This, however, is not what we've been taught. Throughout our lives, in subtle and not-so-subtle ways, society tells us to be careful;

to look before we leap; to make the ten-, twenty-, or thirty-year plan instead of living in the here and now. Action, unless it is the kind of action the Committee approves of, is discouraged. We study and analyze other people's writing, art, photography, movies, music, business acumen, talent. But when it comes time to do these things ourselves, most of us get only as far as the idea. We then allow someone else to write the story, paint the picture, dance the dance, create the product, and produce the movie for us. Hypnotized by the myth of expertise, we live cut off at the head—disconnected from spontaneity, fearful of making mistakes, relieved to allow others to take the risks. Yet, how well does this model serve us? Is it possible it deprives us of the confidence we need to move forward and instead, plants the seeds of procrastination and fear?

## KNOWING BY DOING

Now Act presents a different standpoint, one that advocates *doing in order to know*. The intellect and the Committee despise this action-oriented, spontaneous approach. Before grown-ups teach children to do things "right," children paint, dance, and sing without inhibition. They look at books and pretend they can read. They imagine unlimited possibilities for themselves as explorers, astronauts, ballerinas, circus performers, and presidents. Until society instructs them to take life more seriously and instills the competitive spirit, they think however and whatever they wish. They find the *knowing* in the *doing* by using energy, curiosity, and, yes, even ineptitude. They don't know if their voices are "good" or "bad" or if they can carry a tune, so they sing. They don't care about remembering the steps or being clumsy or making fools of themselves, so they dance. Until we tell them otherwise, making mistakes is part of the fun. However, most adults consider their mistakes to be serious errors, goofs tantamount to sin.

The corruption sets in early in our education when the system begins to process us like some packaged homogenized cheese. Doing things wrong becomes a sin against the authorities. Learning by doing is put aside in favor of doing things right, gaining approval, fitting in. It's no surprise that many of us become perfectionists and procrastinators, constricted by our rigid standards, putting off until tomorrow whatever we can possibly avoid doing today, holding our breath at even the thought of failure.

Knowing by doing is the heart and soul of Now Act. It's the jumping-off point for change and healing, the path to becoming your own authority, and a catalyst for moral action. But how do we choose? What are the doings or actions that bring us into wholeness, that help us discover our truths, release us from enslavement to the Committee, and return us to our blueprints? Moreover, once we know what these actions are, how do we get ourselves to do them?

## KNOWING WHAT TO DO
## AND GETTING YOURSELF TO DO IT

By asking yourself what you want and what's important to you, your path to action becomes clear. For instance:

- What is it you want to know, learn, discover?
- What do you wish to change, heal, find, release, create?
- What gives your life meaning and joy?
- What makes it worth getting out of bed each day?
- Why do you think you are here on this planet, alive in this world?

## READING THE GLYPHS

One day, a woman who has smoked for years and refuses to give it up notices that every cigarette she pulls from her pack is broken.

She decides her problem is that she needs a hardpack. She goes to the store, but the clerk tells her he has none. She goes to another; the story is the same. When she tries to buy a lighter she's told they don't sell them. At this point, she can choose to read the signs that tell her to "break" her habit, or she can insist this experience is random and meaningless.[1]

In this case, she chooses to ignore the message and argues that this is a coincidence. When a friend points out this is a sign, a *glyph*, that favors her quitting—that she might get rid of her constant colds, allergy symptoms, and her hacking cough—she holds a conference with her Committee. The Skeptic doubts that she would benefit at all by stopping at this late date. The Comparer points out that she is special, that she need not follow the herd who have quit smoking. The Blamer labels her friend a member of the Smoke Police, determined to limit her enjoyment and freedom. Quickly, the glyph loses its magic, obscured by the many faces of her false selves.

We introduced glyphs in chapter 4. By revealing, all at once, the meaningful facets of a situation or event, such symbols connect inner with outer and thought with action. Glyphs abound in our daily lives, in our inner world, and in our dreams. But since most of us are in a trance while awake and oblivious while we dream, we often miss them. Yet, once we wake ourselves up and become aware of our intentions and priorities, these signs become more frequent. When we start to respect and to read these glyphs, we become privy to a system of self-direction that flows from our inner wisdom.

Essentially, your glyphs connect you with your intuition, the part of you that naturally knows which action to take and what needs to be changed, worked on, or looked after. Noticing glyphs is a practice of awareness and willingness. What the spiritual master we met in chapter 6 taught still holds: "The secret of life is paying attention." There is no glyph expert to do this for you. When you take advantage of this way of knowing, you become the Watcher: calm, centered, relaxed, concentrating without effort on the little things in daily life. As you go about your business, you *observe* the sensations in your body, *notice* your thoughts and images, and *undo* the Committee's debilitating refrain.

## BECOME YOUR OWN GLYPHOLOGIST

It's fun to become your own glyphologist. It makes life interesting and meaningful.

Think about the following occurrences:

- The chocolate cake you are about to eat, for no good reason, falls off your fork and lands on your lap.

Might this be telling you that this is where the cake will eventually wind up—on your body as well as inside it?

- You trip or fall while on your way somewhere.

Think about what's been tripping you up lately. Or where it is that you don't really want (or need) to go.

- Something or someone appears unexpectedly (or unusually often).

What unfinished business do you have with this person?

- You misplace your appointment book that lists your busy schedule.

Do you need a day off, or some unstructured time?

- You wake up and your shoulder and back ache.

What burden are you shouldering that's painful for you to bear?

We often mistake these events for accidents or random occurrences. Actually, they are signs and point out a pattern that tells you about yourself, your life, and your relationship to the world. They are an integral part of life and living. Once you get good at this, you begin to realize that no matter what happens, everything is really all right.[2]

## SIX SIMPLE ACTION INDICATORS: KNOWING WHAT TO DO

Once you make it your intention to Now Act, six action indicators will serve as beacons for you. Paying attention to these items will give you clues about how to act and which direction to take. Action indicators include (but certainly are not limited to):

1. *Glyphs*. These signs appear spontaneously and can indicate the best direction in which to go.
2. *Imagery*. Your imagery reveals who you are and directs you toward choosing your actions in the world.
3. *Prayer*. Asking for guidance in doing instead of asking that something be done *for* you will help you Now Act.
4. *Dreams*. Dreams reveal the actions that best serve you and others, and they refer you to the meaning and purpose of your own life.
5. *A Moral Code*. Your moral code may be the Ten Commandments, which are ancient laws that impose discipline but also foster freedom. Or you may, like the Dalai Lama, follow the code of kindness at all times and act with compassion, empathy, and love. A moral code is a framework that connects those who use it with their source. When you don't know what action to take, your moral code, whatever it may be, serves as a guide.

6. *Everyday Life*. At any given moment you may get a strong feeling about something. A felt sense, an image, or a thought may instantly pop into your mind. If you don't honor these, they quickly pass. Such moments may prompt you to take immediate action or may present you with a future option. Either way, everyday life is an endless source of opportunities to Now Act.

## Overthrowing the Tyrant

Jan had lived in her cooperative apartment in New York for about a year when she first heard stories about the board president's scare-tactic politics. Initially, she thought of it as gossip but soon discovered that the issue went deeper than a mere personality conflict. Some of the older tenants were frightened. It shocked her that in this small, quiet building, one man wielded the power to create an atmosphere of subservience and fear. Jan became more attentive to the remarks of neighbors, to the attitudes of the staff, and to her own experiences with this person whose manner was imperious and rude.

When some of her neighbors asked that she try to unseat the tyrant by running for the board herself, Jan hesitated. She saw herself as the new kid on the block and preferred that someone else step forward, but no one was willing. Instead, residents offered stories of this man's venomous ways and warned that he would retaliate against his opponent. When Jan asked what form this retaliation might take, they murmured about nasty confrontations and threatening letters. Jan ordinarily shied away from confrontation, since it seemed to trigger asthmatic symptoms, but this man's behavior was so outrageous that she decided to run. For Jan, this was a spiritual turning point—one where she chose to go beyond self-interest and to link her quest for freedom and healing to the world at large. It was reading the glyphs, attending to prayer and imagery, and following her moral code that directed and facilitated Jan's actions.

On the night of the annual board meeting, the tyrant was in his glory, working the room like a practiced politician while Jan's Committee was out in full force. They told her she was foolish, out of her league, and that this man had it "all sewn up." Noticing some constriction in her chest, Jan adjourned the Committee by focusing on the task at hand. As she stood and introduced herself to the group, the tightness was transformed, becoming instead a sense of excitement and liberation. She realized that doing what was unfamiliar and out of character was not going to kill her. It actually felt good.

Until this time, Jan's work with this program had focused on her inner life, her relationships with family, with friends, and with the asthma. Deciding to oppose the tyrant transformed her desire to become free into an active presence in the world. It expanded her perception of healing to include right relationship within her community. It Undid Jan's belief that she was nonpolitical, that others knew more, were braver and better suited to this task than she. Her involvement in the election, *without concern for the outcome*, made her into a soldier of truth. When she stood up for what she believed was right and announced her willingness to run, she bore witness to the importance of justice and goodness as part of the moral order. Once she stated aloud, "I am Jan," she vanquished fear and doubt.

> Saying who we are should not be taken for granted. To finish the sentence that begins with "*I am* . . ." is to emulate God and to stand for something godly. Announcing our name is a transcendent act that should dispel all surprise and doubt about the goodness of the universe.[3]

Some of the imagery Jan used to see herself through this difficult time included "The Triple Mirror" and "Liberation from Slavery," both of which we include here. The first enabled her to see herself creating these new actions; the second generated a sense of freedom from her fear and from the asthma.

## THE TRIPLE MIRROR[4]

*Intention:* To create change and growth. To generate action and healing.

*Frequency:* Once a day for 21 days for less than three minutes. Stop for seven days. Then, if you wish, do another 21-day cycle.

Close your eyes and breathe out three times. See yourself standing before a triple mirror, the kind you find in the dressing room of a store. Look at yourself in the mirror on your left. See the way you are now. Breathe out one time and look at yourself in the mirror in the center. See the way you want to be (or what you want to be doing) in one to three weeks (or months) from now. Breathe out one time and look at yourself in the mirror on your right. See the way you want to be when you have completed this action and are in full bloom. Then breathe out and open your eyes.

*Note: If you are left-handed, reverse the process and make the mirror on the right your starting point (the present).*

## LIBERATION FROM SLAVERY[5]✷

*Intention:* To generate taking action. To free yourself emotionally and physically from asthma.

*Frequency:* Once a day, in the morning, for 21 days, for up to three minutes.

Close your eyes and breathe out three times. See before you the image of your difficulty, disease, or pain. See the chains that bind you together. Know that this difficulty has created a life of its own. See and feel how you are a slave to this life of darkness. Breathe out one time. Find a way to unlock or to break these chains and

release yourself from bondage. Do this now. As the chains fall
away, take your first steps in the direction of freedom and truth.
What happens? How do you feel? Then breathe out and open your
eyes.

*Note: Over the next 21 days, your images may change. There's no
need to resist this change. It's part of the process. Remember that as your
images change, so do your beliefs and your physiology.*

## KNOWING WHAT NOT TO DO:
## FOUR FALSE-ACTION INDICATORS

What is not valuable are the messages of the Committee. Although
these directives may seem enticing, they provoke anxiety and guilt
and include the following:[6]

1. Obey the "shoulds" and "musts." I should follow my doctor's
   (wife's, mother's, friend's) advice, even when it goes against
   my own beliefs.
2. Live by the "Crystal Ball Chronicles," also known as "If-Then
   Scenarios." If I run/jog without carrying my inhaler, I might
   have an attack.
3. Follow social standards. Everyone else uses regular medication
   for asthma symptoms, so I'll look foolish if I try imagery.
4. Seek recognition. By following my doctor's advice, she will
   like and admire me.

These false-action indicators hold particular danger for asthmatics. Maggie's story illustrates how easily we fall prey to them.

## Learning on the Job

Maggie, an asthmatic since early childhood, works at a job she dislikes in a city she wants to leave. Recently her supervisor confronted her with negative feedback from her colleagues, and Maggie felt hurt and betrayed. Immediately, her Committee chastised her for her imperfections and her failure to live up to its standards. It demanded to know how she could be liked, respected, and regarded as an important player on the team when her supervisor and colleagues found fault with her. The Committee insisted that she get the full story. They demanded that she ask, "Who said these things?" "When were these remarks made?" "Why tell me now?" But Maggie's Committee misled her. The issue was not who said what; such commentary only fed her insecurities and added more weight to the drama. The point was, and continues to be, her need to release her fear and stand up for herself.

The supervisor's gripe is like the telephone game we played when we were kids. The first person whispers something in the next person's ear, and one by one the information gets passed along until we finally hear the jumble it turns into at the other end of the line. It's interesting that a synonym for *gripe* is *hang up*. Maggie could read the glyph of the gripe and "hang up" on the discussion. In order to do this, she becomes the Watcher: she separates herself from the Committee and creates enough space to recognize that what it's telling her is false. The next step is to form an image, like hanging up the phone or, better still, hanging up the supervisor (putting him "out to dry" on a clothesline might be fun). The process is analogous to using homeopathy, where you treat like with like.

Maggie might Now Act in other ways. Instead of engaging in defensive dialogue, she could choose to walk out of the room. The shock of such an action might silence the supervisor and transform the whole situation. Yet Maggie's fear of losing her job prevents her from doing this. It is the same fear and uncertainty that keeps her from moving to a new place while making up a story about a future outcome that ensures her enslavement.

## Maggie's Dream: A True and Valuable Action Indicator

That night, Maggie dreams that she's pulled over by the police. When their dogs search her car, a bag of heroin turns up in the backseat. She feels set up and begs them not to arrest her, explaining how this would ruin her career. Her pleas fall on deaf ears. The officer tells her that she's in possession of an illegal substance and is holding enough to be charged with suspicion of drug trafficking. Maggie begins sobbing. Then she wakes up.

Unlike the voice of the Committee, Maggie's dream tells the truth. It's her personal mirror and a genuine indicator for a way in which she might Now Act. Being pulled over reveals that she has been sidetracked (pulled off the road, her path) by the authorities (in this case the police). At work she feels derailed by the supervisor, the company rules, the job. In the dream she feels victimized, frightened of losing her reputation and career. She pleads with the authorities and protests her innocence. But the more she implores these authority figures, the more anxious she becomes. This is analogous to the situation at work, where she also feels victimized and afraid. Her error with the dream police is the same as her error with her supervisor. Both of these authority figures undermine her confidence and sap her will.

## Maggie's Personal Dream Medicine

The dream, however, holds the key to freedom. Just as the difficulty with her supervisor provides Maggie with a catalyst to change her stance, so does the heroin. As the central dream image, it has more than just the obvious meaning of addiction, escape, and criminality. On one level, Maggie is addicted to approval, longs to escape the restrictions of her job, and feels like a criminal who has done something wrong, but all she need do is add one more letter to the word *heroin* to transform herself from victim to victor—or from victim to Heroin(e).

Overall, the dream advised her to Undo her habit of bowing down to authorities—a violation of the Ten Commandments (her moral code), which forbids idol worship. Instead of denying the existence of the Heroine (and the heroin) in her life, she might turn toward these qualities of courage and addiction and thus own them. Maggie needed to liberate herself by weeding out the belief she was a victim. To do this, she had to recognize the connection between the asthma and her addiction to recognition and approval.

By thinking of her job as a stepping-stone instead of allowing it to constrict and diminish her, Maggie began to seek out simple ways to act heroic. Once she recognized both her *heroin* and her *heroine* qualities, her perspective shifted. Within two months of having this dream, she had left her job and reinvented her career. For the first time in years, she began to have fun and to breathe without wheezing. To aid her in her efforts to take these actions, Maggie used the following imagery exercise:

---

## THE HERO OR HEROINE[7]

*Intention:* To generate energy for taking action, and to eliminate any obstacles.

*Frequency:* Once a day for 21 days, for no longer than two minutes. May also use as an on-the-spot action generator whenever needed.

Close your eyes and breathe out three times. See and sense yourself become your own hero or heroine. Notice how you look. Feel the powerful energy you generate. Trust this energy as it flows through you and around you, revitalizing your body and mind. See before you any obstacle that is blocking your way. Knowing that there are no limitations in the imagination, find a way to overcome this obstacle. Do this now. See how you feel and what happens. Then breathe out and open your eyes.

# FIVE ACTION GENERATORS:
# GETTING YOURSELF TO DO IT

The leap between knowing what to do and getting yourself to do it can seem insurmountable. The following action generators facilitate this leap and even make it FUN. For those of you who habitually procrastinate, the next few pages can change your life. This list of action generators includes several ideas already mentioned as action indicators; we use them here with a different intention. We discuss each of them in greater depth below.

1. *Humor.* Taking things seriously makes them seem more important. The more important things seem, the more we ponder them and the less apt we are to "just do it." Humor generates a way of looking at life that lightens things up. Feeling lighter frees you to move (take action) more easily.

2. *A Prayer Collage.* With this collage technique you create a pattern of positive images that help generate your return to health. It's a valuable action tool for children as well as adults.

3. *Music.* Music moves us, both inside and out. It accompanies us throughout life as we celebrate birthdays, fall in love, walk down the aisle, join the parade, march into battle, and mourn. What could be more effective for creating spontaneous movement in life? Your task is to listen and use what you hear for moving forward.

4. *Imagery.* When you change your image, you change your belief. Movement and change on the inside trigger the same on the outside.

5. *Kindness.* Kindness breaks through the regrets and resentments that keep anger (and breath) locked inside us. Being generous and considerate to yourself and others initiates flow and movement in your life.

## HUMOR: THE ANTIDOTE TO ALL ILLS

What is the payoff if we take life seriously? Who besides the Committee finds this so important? Certainly not Norman Cousins, who in *Anatomy of an Illness* recounted his recovery from a condition his doctors advised was fatal. Cousins, then publisher of *Saturday Review*, was among the first people who gave public voice to humor as the emotional catalyst for recovery. The laughs he got from vintage Marx Brothers films and old reruns of *Candid Camera* in conjunction with megadoses of vitamin C succeeded where conventional medicine had failed. To the amazement of his doctors and the scientific community, he reversed his cellular disease.[8]

The *New England Journal of Medicine* gave an extraordinary response to Cousins's original article about his recovery. Medical journals reprinted it, medical schools included it in course materials, thousands of physicians from all over the world wrote him letters of praise, and Cousins was sought out as a speaker in medical schools throughout the country. His experience became legendary, and he later joined the faculty of the UCLA Medical School.[9]

### The Dynamic Duo: Science and Fun

Dr. Hunter D. Adams, better known as Patch, was another early proponent of humor. Dr. Adams, who calls humor "an antidote to all ills," has never walked the conventional path. Even in medical school, he infuriated his teachers by questioning their judgments and dressing up as a clown to make his patients laugh. From the beginning, Adams has been a doer, a true activist for compassionate medicine who sees humor as the great healer and chooses to do his "clowning wherever the suffering is great."[10]

Adams believes in the restorative power of compassion, love, and laughter—qualities he sees sorely missing in modern medicine, with its "doctor-patient emotional void." To him, the most serious illness afflicting today's world is neither cancer nor AIDS but greed.[11] His Gesundheit Institute in West Virginia treats patients, not only with conventional medication, but with humor and love, all at no charge. Patch Adams is definitely on the fringe. Not many of us go to the store wearing our underwear on the outside of our clothes, entertain hospitalized children in Russia, or have movies made about our lives. This is the type of behavior the Committee finds outrageous. After all, what kind of doctor could Adams be—treating his patients with emotional support and humorous entertainment instead of "real" medicine!

But Adams isn't alone in his lighthearted attitude. Even "serious" scientists can be playful. For example, Sir Roger Penrose, Oxford professor, mathematician, physicist, author, and one of the greatest living disciples of Albert Einstein, keeps toys in his office! Penrose claims, "Science and fun cannot be separated."[12] For Cousins, Adams, and Penrose, humor is a staple in life, not something to be brought out of the closet and polished up on special occasions. They show us how cultivating a humorous outlook can help to reverse the Committee's decree that we take life seriously. This shift leaves us room for error, for making fools of ourselves, for *learning by doing*. Playing the fool is not the disaster your Committee would have you believe. Synonyms for *fool* include *booby, ninny, bozo, yahoo,* and *clown.* What fun! How liberating and delightful not to care what people think: to trip over yourself and laugh; to sing off-key; to dance and miss the beat. This attitude is reminiscent of the old adage about angels—that they can fly because they take themselves lightly. We too can transform by taking ourselves lightly. We have only to put on our imaginal humor glasses and perceive life less seriously to find merriment in our ordinary experiences, and even to indulge in some old-fashioned buffoonery.

## A Merry Heart Makes Breathing Easier

Have you ever been admonished for thinking something was funny, for acting silly, for not taking things seriously enough? As a child, did adults (parents, teachers) tell you to "wipe that smile off your face"? Have you experienced that out-of-control feeling when the smile becomes even wider and you burst out laughing? Patch Adams preferred being light to heavy, humorous to serious. He defied the medical establishment and made this his way of life. How many of us have the courage to live our own truth and disregard the norm? How often do you smile, laugh, have fun? What happens to your breathing when you act this way?

Medical researchers throughout the country have studied the effects of laughter on the body. Among the many benefits they cite is enhanced respiration.[13] Your Committee may hate to hear this, but *laughter contributes to good health*, particularly for people with asthma. Scientific evidence is fast accumulating in support of the biblical saying "A merry heart doeth good like a medicine."[14] Humorist Mel Brooks, comedian, producer, actor, and physician of FUN wisdom, has this to say: "Humor keeps you rolling along, singing a song. When you laugh, it's an explosion of the lungs. You laugh, you breathe, the blood runs, and everything is circulating."[15] As for crying, the good doctor says, "You feel happier when you're laughing than crying—unless you're crying with happiness."

## All About Harry

Harry had been asthmatic since his early twenties. At the age of fifty-six, he made a "serious" commitment to find a new way to deal with it. Being serious was nothing new for Harry. He was born serious—his baby pictures proved it—and he had remained serious his entire life. When he read a newspaper, Harry took each disastrous article to heart. In his law practice, he approached the problems of his clients as if they were his own. Even his daughter's light case of acne kept a smile from his face.

Harry's fiancée felt the seriousness had gone too far and was casting a pall on their relationship. She suggested that he lighten up. At work one day, a colleague handed Harry an old-fashioned joke book. As he read it, Harry began to chuckle. The more he laughed, the more he enjoyed himself, and the better he felt. Soon he came up with the idea to call his fiancée every day with a new joke. Despite her personal disinterest in joke telling, the fiancée applauded his decision. As a surprise bonus, she began to enjoy the daily phone jokes. They made her laugh out loud, and from then on the relationship took on a more lighthearted tone. You too can create conscious humor in your life. Just do the following:

---

## CLOWNING AROUND

*Intention:* To laugh, have fun, lighten up.

*Frequency:* Do at least three of these, once a day, every day of your life.

Laugh or smile at least three times to begin the day.

Tell a joke to a friend.

Do something silly.

Watch something funny enough to make you laugh out loud.

Skip down the street.

Make fun of yourself.

Add to these whatever you personally find humorous.

---

## Not Alone

This ritual of a joke a day gave Harry an opening for other aspects of himself to emerge. As with Cousins, the laughter did not occur in isolation. It was part of the range of positive thoughts and emotions that stimulate joy and healing, including a sense of possibility, faith, love, purpose, meaning, hope, merriment, and the will to live. Harry's life became lighter, more spontaneous, less serious. His breathing became easier, freer. At last, Harry was having FUN.

But how can this be? you might ask. How can a simple action like telling jokes make such a difference? On the other hand, how can this *not* be? When life comes together in harmonious and healing ways, why do we say "I can't believe it" or "It's too good to be true"? After all, we seem to find it ordinary, run of the mill, when things *don't* work out. Indeed, it is unnatural and strange for serendipity and synchronicity to be absent. It's then that we know we are not attuned to the flow of life. When we renounce our habits and live in the present moment, even things as practical and simple as Harry's joke book can open up our lives as if by magic.

What's more, a sense of humor is not an inborn personality trait that we either have or we don't. According to researcher Michelle Newman, an affiliate professor and senior research associate at the University of Pennsylvania department of psychology, "It's a coping tool that can be taught." People can learn to look on the brighter side of things, and the effects are similar to exercise in athletes, prompting the production of endorphins and lessening stress hormones.[16] With a turn of mind and a change of heart, miracles are possible.

The next technique for generating action furthers the light-hearted outlook we have just discussed. This special process was suggested by an extraordinary woman who teaches how it's possible to create a bridge to the divine through the simplest of processes. If it's a miracle you are looking for, this might just be the way to create one.

## A PRAYER MADE OF PICTURES

Have you ever looked at a photograph of yourself taken at a time of great happiness and had a sense memory of that experience? Colette Aboulker-Muscat of Jerusalem, a renowned mystic and teacher, has a reputation for remarkable clarity of mind and great wisdom. Her repertoire includes many creative and playful healing techniques. One of these uses collage to create a change in outlook. Making this involves combining personal photographs along with other items and treasured mementos that for you represent happiness and health. Such a picture elicits an optimistic response and promotes healing. The process of creating what we call a Prayer Collage becomes an analogy for creating a new and joyful life; it offers a concrete image of the way that you want to see yourself in the world.

For Maggie, our heroine, this process proved life changing. "As I looked at myself running, smiling, and laughing, I experienced a bodily sensation of being able to do this again," she told us. "Yet, as wonderful as this process was," Maggie added, "it demanded that I persevere and take even the smallest action each day. It motivated me to clean the house of old stuff that kept me tied to the past, an action that left a space, not only in my home, but inside myself. Before I worked with the FUN program, I might have identified this space as a sensation of emptiness. Now I refrained from giving it a label. Above all, it gave me a way to release my old life—the one I had planned on living—so that my new life might finally begin."

## CREATE A PRAYER COLLAGE

*Intention:* To create a new and joyful life.

*Frequency:* Do once. Then add to or change at any time.

Gather pictures of yourself and mementos that give you a feeling of happiness and optimism.

Arrange these on a large piece of paper in a manner that pleases you.

Paste or tape them so that you can rearrange them as often as you wish.

Place the collage where it can act as a constant reminder of the way that you want to be.

Add whatever new items strike your fancy, or remove whatever no longer pleases you.

When you make your collage, your Committee may try to limit you, telling you what's possible and what's not. But this is *your* picture, *your* truth, not theirs. Be your own authority. Tell any unbidden advisers (including Committee members, parents, friends, medical "experts") they need not apply. Listening to their pronouncements devalues the worth of your creation and plants insidious nocebos. This process is between you and God or whatever Higher Power or universal energy you believe in or choose to trust. Change these images as often as you wish. See what happens. Enjoy!

The Prayer Collage creates a concrete image of yourself as you want to be. By selecting these elements and putting them together, you turn yourself toward physical, emotional, and spiritual change. The next section of this chapter furthers this transition.

## IF MUSIC BE THE SOUND OF ACTION, PLAY ON

While imagery turns our senses inward, music functions on a dual level—attuning us to the physical world of action as well as to the inner world of feeling. Music presents us with a simple yet powerful method of going beyond the logical mind, dispensing with the Committee, and taking action in life each day. We break the chains to the past as we sense its rhythm and breathe in unison. We listen to the words, and our lives unfold before us. We hear the melody, and it opens our hearts. In the previous chapter on Undoing, we suggested that you create a healing tape. Here, you embellish this tape however you wish. Then we suggest that you employ the power of this music as a call to action. The music you listen to, play, create, sing, and move to is a personal resource that connects you with the divine source. Allow it to lead you. And through its grace, generate a sense of balance, tempo, and harmony in your everyday life.[17]

## DEFINING OURSELVES BY OUR ACTIONS

We may think complex thoughts, feel passionate emotions, and compose endless daydreams about what we might become, but it's

our actions that render our living image. Whether we are kind or
mean-spirited, spontaneous or analytical, selfish or caring defines us
as human beings. It's what we *do* and how we behave that manifests
our beliefs and determines our presence in the world. Through
even the most subtle manner and deed, we draw people to us or
turn them away. Our actions may create peace or turmoil, engender
a gathering together or a splitting apart, both within ourselves and
with those around us.

## Simple Acts of Kindness

Alan pursued Caroline tenaciously when they first met. But
though she found him attractive, generous, and personable, she
resisted him. Then one evening he spoke of the recent loss of his
father. In a quiet voice, Alan confided how he had held his
father's hand as he lay dying, reassuring him he was not alone,
remaining beside him until he breathed his last breath. At that
moment, Caroline's heart opened; she envisioned the scene so
clearly, it took her breath away. With her own parents, she had
been unable to do this. For her, this act of kindness, this gracious-
ness of the heart, instantly defined Alan as someone she wanted
to know better—and revealed qualities she wanted to cultivate in
herself.

What actions define you as a person? In what ways do you shine
*your* light into the world? When Aldous Huxley, one of the twenti-
eth century's great thinkers, was asked what he thought was most
important for living a spiritual life, he answered simply: "Just to be a
little kinder." Acts of kindness go a long way toward creating grace in
our lives. And these acts may be directed toward ourselves as well as
toward others. In the ancient book *Sayings of the Fathers,* in which
rabbis and scholars of many generations comment on the ethics and
morality necessary for creating a decent civilization, it says:

> If I am not for me, who will be for me?
> If I am only for myself, what am I?

Cheryl, whom we met in chapter 4, wanted to repair her relationship with her grandmother, even though she had been gone for thirty years. After discovering where she was buried, Cheryl visited the grave. As she stood beside the untended grave, the guilt and anger buried inside her rose to the surface. Through her tears, she recalled her mother's cruel treatment of this woman and, worse, her own insensitivity. Cheryl asked her grandmother's forgiveness and acknowledged that it was time for the family to release the past. In her journal she wrote:

> Grandma, it's time for healing. Sometimes we can't understand why things happen, they seem so unfair. We can only try to learn, to keep our hearts open and to find joy in each day's existence on earth. ... We can change the world by spreading kindness and understanding. God, please help me dissipate this anger. Maybe I can bury it here and leave it.

As Cheryl observed, to find joy in each day's existence, to spread kindness and understanding, liberates and heals us. The asthma epidemic is a glyph for the ills of the world. It informs us that we have shirked our role as caretakers—of the earth, ourselves, one another. As we destroy the environment, cutting down forests and polluting the air and water, the earth loses its power to breathe and defend itself, just as we do. To resuscitate the earth and yourself, to restore your breath, and to renew both personal and universal resources, you may want to practice these acts:

*Do unto Others*
- Recycle with the intention of rejuvenating the earth.
- Write a letter (or call) someone who lives alone or is ill.
- Offer a helping hand to an infirm or elderly person who is crossing a street.
- Invite a friend for tea even if you think he or she should invite you.

- Visit an animal shelter and adopt a pet.
- Pay more loving attention to the pets you already have.
- Donate something that you do not use but have been holding on to.
- Pick up some litter (even if *you* didn't drop it).
- Volunteer.

No kindness is insignificant. Your body rejoices and heals when you go beyond self-involvement and act with generosity and care. Just remember that you must balance these altruistic acts toward the earth and others with similar acts of kindness toward yourself. Here are some ideas for practicing kindness toward yourself:

*Do unto Yourself*
- Get a great haircut.
- Visit a museum.
- Drink juice or water from a crystal goblet instead of your regular glass.
- Read a novel that sizzles with your kind of sizzle, whatever that is.
- Imagine at least three wonderful things before breakfast.
- Laugh a lot.
- Make love.
- Study yoga.
- Walk down a new street.

Acts of kindness abound when you are open to them. Begin with the choices life offers you. Jan confronts the tyrant and overthrows him in the election; Maggie unhinges the Committee and becomes her own heroine; Cheryl visits her grandmother's grave and makes amends; Caroline opens her heart and gets to know Alan. All act in their own time, in their own way, and manage to set things moving in themselves and in the world. The methods for facilitating action that we have shared in this chapter can light your creative spark and fuel the will necessary for moving forward.

Manifesting whatever it is that you want in life is the result of taking action. The next imagery exercise will help you with this. Earlier in the chapter, Jan used "The Triple Mirror" and "Liberation from Slavery" to overthrow the tyrant. Here you have the opportunity to stop *wishing* and to start creating through using the active process of imagery.

---

### THE GOLDEN NET [18]

*Intention:* To manifest what you want and need in your life.

*Frequency:* Once a day for 21 days, for one to two minutes each day. Or as needed, whenever you feel stuck.

Close your eyes and breathe out three times. See yourself going to the ocean. Once you are there, cast out your golden nets. Cast them as far and wide as your imagination takes them. Let go of all your limitations. As you draw your nets back in, see that they are returning to you with all you want, need, and desire. Then open your eyes.

---

Now Act completes the third part of the FUN program. Take time now to read the following essentials before going on to chapter 9.

*The Essentials of Now Act*
1. *Act Now.* Don't postpone for the "right time." Remember, the word *Act* is preceded by *Now*, not *Know!*
2. *Clarify your intention.* Hold it clearly in your mind, and begin.
3. *Maintain your integrity.* Align your intentions with your moral code. Do not compromise yourself or others.

4. *Ask, "How can I use this?"* Use whatever arises as an opportunity for change. Read the discomfort as messages, the irritations as clues, and the obstacles as challenges.
5. *Go beyond your personal concerns.* Become connected and involved. Shine your light into the world even in simple ways.
6. *Learn by living.* Be your own authority. Do in order to know!
7. *Practice kindness* with yourself and others.

### CHAPTER 9

# TURNING WORK INTO PLAY

## Mind Medicine to Empower Children

*The potential possibilities of any child are the most intriguing in all creation.*

RAY L. WILBUR

Most children are natural FUNsters. Kids delight in imagery, drawing, music, and humor. This kind of medicine suits them just fine. We suggest that children try all these techniques, though it's imagery we find most effective. The reason for this is simple: kids find it easy to gain access to beliefs that transport and transform themselves and their circumstances. When young children watch mimes or puppets, they truly believe that the mime is eating or climbing a ladder or throwing a ball. The invisible exists without question; it doesn't matter that it can't be seen. For them, puppets are extraordinary beings, not just hollow fabric and plaster, held aloft by the hands of human puppeteers. The same phenomenon occurs when children practice imagery. They suspend disbelief. What they see is what they believe and vice versa. If no one disparages their efforts, using a golden inhaler is easy for them. It's also nonaddictive, playful, and immediately available at all times.

Mind medicine for kids shows them it's possible to become personally empowered. They learn to know and respect themselves despite any illness. This chapter gives you more than an array of techniques you can use with children: it offers a perspective on children's increasing susceptibility and suggests ways to address childhood asthma by other than the ordinary, pharmacological means. For those parents wary of taking children off medication, there is no need to think of this program as an either-or approach. We suggest that you offer these techniques to your kids with no strings attached. Many children are able to wean themselves from conventional medication with this quite naturally. Some lessen their medication considerably. Still others experience a complete and rapid healing. There is no norm. At the very least, children who use these techniques can get a better sense of themselves— feel more powerful, safer, more relaxed, joyful, and free. The following example shares how one child's use of imagery relieved her symptoms and enabled her to deal with some stressful events in her family.

Helen is seven and has been asthmatic since she was twenty months old. She uses a nonsteroidal inhaler and has tried homeopathy, acupuncture, and herbal remedies, all with some success. But though these treatments have helped, they haven't eliminated her problem. The asthma recurs most often when she is overtired or upset.

Helen's parents have been unhappy in their marriage for years and are considering divorce. Although they have not offered Helen any details regarding their possible separation, she's aware that "something is going on." In fact, Helen's parents have *never* been happy together. And though they remain bound by their mutual history and family business, the union lacks joy. Even before Helen was born, tension and regret existed. Recently, it's become much worse. One night, after she hears her parents arguing, Helen begins to cough; she feels nervous and upset. To get some quick relief, she uses her inhaler. As we have pointed out, grieving and loss are important elements in relation to asthma. And Helen seems to know a lot more about all this than she is willing to say.

Helen's mom has used imagery for symptoms of her own successfully and believes it can give her daughter a way to control the asthma. She also thinks it can help Helen express what's going on emotionally. The imagery exercise Helen uses, called "Box of Balloons," is one that children (and adults) enjoy. She enters a room, finds a box containing balloons of many colors, selects a blue one, blows it up, and ties it off with a string. Helen imagines going outside while holding tightly to the string and floating with the balloon, high above the earth, until she reaches a farm. There she sees a stable; inside she finds a brown horse that she decides to ride. Though she has never ridden before, she has no fear of saddling up the horse, mounting it, and riding around the farm. She feels happy; she is having FUN. Helen then uses this exercise to start each day, knowing that every time she rides the brown horse she leaves the asthma and unhappiness behind. After 21 days of doing this, she reports that she has not needed to use the inhaler and now plans to take riding lessons.

Riding the horse gives Helen a way to release her tension while freeing her breath. But all does not stop here. For Helen to continue healing on a deeper level, her parents must liberate themselves from the emotional limbo that generates so much distress and anxiety in the family. To accomplish this, they need to choose whether to leave the marriage or to make a go of it, thus setting everyone free to move on. Try this exercise with your own child now. Whether or not your child has asthma, it's a good way to have some FUN.

## BOX OF BALLOONS[1]

*Intention:* To create a sense of freedom and relaxation. To relieve the asthma.

*Frequency:* For 21 days if you find something you want. Or whenever feeling pressured or constricted by symptoms or circumstances, for up to three minutes.

Close your eyes and breathe out three times. Imagine you are standing in front of a table. On the table is a box. Open it and see that inside are balloons of different colors. Choose one of any color. Blow it up to its full size. Tie it with a golden string; hold onto it, and don't let go. Now see it rising above your head. Go outside into a garden or a meadow and, holding onto the balloon, see yourself rising into the air above you. Have some FUN while floating around out there. Know that you can go anywhere you want to go and do anything you want to do. See what happens. Then breathe out and open your eyes.

## SOLVING THE ASTHMA PUZZLE

Young asthmatics like Helen are not uncommon. Since 1980, asthma has increased by 160 percent among children in America[2] and has become the number one cause of hospitalization and school absenteeism.[3] The risk of asthma has soared, even in areas where pollution is minimal or nonexistent. No one can fully explain this. Some experts blame environmental pollution, the ozone layer, or poor nutrition. Others fault technology: television, computers, sealed rooms. A growing number cite an irresponsible use of medications: antibiotics, vaccines, steroids—drugs that disable and destroy the natural functions of the immune system. Parents of asthmatics feel confused, guilty, and powerless. They want to regain control. It is unbearable for parents to see their children suffer while knowing that prevention and healing of this suffering is beyond their reach.

In the 1970s, children left home to live in hospital-run facilities in the belief that "parentectomy" was the answer. Later, experts dropped this guilt-provoking idea. In the new psychological jargon, the family is "the solution, not the problem." Parents are invited to become involved in their child's treatment through becoming familiar with medicines, with the use of inhalers, and with peak flow monitors (used to measure exhalation and monitor possible attacks). No invitation is extended, however, to look at their children's experience from the mindbody perspective. Though stress might be mentioned, it's viewed as something to avoid, defuse— never directly addressed or discussed.

One of the more recent and popular theories proposes that asthma is an immune system malfunction related to an overproduction of Immunoglobulin E (IgE),[4] the antibody that protects our bodies from parasites. This has inclined science to classify asthma as a *chemical* imbalance. In response to this, research has turned toward pharmacological means to block and prevent allergic inflammation, thus spawning even more drug dependency for asthmatics.

However, genuine healing looks toward balancing the organism itself, not just blocking the allergic response. From a mindbody perspective, inflammation represents anger. We feel *inflamed, boil over*, get *hot under the collar*. This makes perfect sense when we recall, as mentioned in chapter 5, that *wheeze* comes from the Old Norse root meaning "to hiss"; yet when we release our anger, the body regains equilibrium and restores itself to harmony. With this more integrated viewpoint, we focus on the symptom as bearing some value. We stop asking what *causes* asthma, and we search instead for the correspondences, the connections and relationships. With regard to children, these primary relationships involve families, schools, friends, and communities.

## Children at Risk

Regardless of the other factors at play, science uses the genetic component as a strong marker for the likelihood of developing asthma. But research has established that genetic risk is not an isolated circumstance[5]—that "disruptive situations" or intense stress, such as death, job loss, or divorce, substantially increase the probability of asthma in the child. A recent study in New York City showed an exceptionally high rate of asthma among homeless children: 38 percent, double the rate found in some of the city's poorest neighborhoods and six times the national rate. Dr. Suzanne Hurd, director of the division of lung diseases at the National Heart, Lung, and Blood Institute, said that even though poor children in big cities are disproportionately affected, she found these "terribly high rates" among homeless children surprising.[6]

The economic deprivation of poverty alone can't explain this. Since homeless children have twice as much asthma as other kids in poverty circumstances, might this not tell us that it's the trauma of becoming homeless that lies at the core? Isn't it possible that losing a home, a familiar environment, and being constantly shuttled from place to place engender grieving great enough to irritate and inflame the lungs (the organ most closely related to the place of joy within us)? We could look at the asthma statistic as a natural correspondence, an exquisite mirror reflecting the event and the process of childhood homelessness.

A study conducted by Dr. David Mrazek, Chief of Psychiatry and Behavioral Sciences at Children's National Medical Center in Washington, D.C., makes a stunning case for the emotional well-being of the family as a criterion to predict which children will get asthma. Interestingly, the study revealed that situations occurring even *before* birth are important determinants. According to Mrazek's statistics, wheezing is far more likely to begin by the age of two if stress occurs in the year *before* the child's birth, especially when this stress continues during infancy.[7]

What could be worse than seeing our children helpless, unable to breathe? Even the slightest thought that we, as parents, may in any way be responsible for this phenomenon is intolerable. The studies and statistics mentioned here are not meant as accusations. Shame, blame, and laying guilt lead us into darkness and have no place in the FUN approach. It's clear that our children's pain tears us apart and that pointing a finger doesn't help. What is integral to healing our children and ourselves is acknowledging the relationship of all that goes on in our lives. We can look not just to outside events and to the environment, but to one another—to our loves and hates, gains and losses, grief and joy; this is the mindbody stance. Once we recognize this tapestry of relationship that we weave, we can then begin to make those changes that create new patterns, that foster emotional health and an asthma-free life.

## The Window of Vulnerability

The first few years of life may be "a window of vulnerability," a critical time in the development of asthma whether or not genetic risk is a factor. Studies like Mrazek's clearly show that early emotional relationships are as important as genetics, pollution, allergens, foods, and viral respiratory diseases. It seems that *all* these triggers, both physical and mental can sensitize children's airways and turn a genetic predisposition into a reality. However, mindbody medicine finds, time and again, that asthma first appears and recurs, not from a specific cause but in correspondence to a confluence of events, emotions, issues, and relationships.

We are a people fascinated by genetics. It offers the perfect arena for analyzing *why:* why we get a particular disease, why we live to a certain age, why we have a specific IQ. Genetics provides us with an identity, a label. The Blamer on our Committee loves it since it abdicates personal responsibility for any of our shortcomings. We cite genetics as the immutable factor and blame our problem on heredity. In a society that romances the victim mentality, this is an excellent fit. But what happens to our sense of wholeness, choice, and power when we worship at the altar of genetic science?

The theory of genetic makeup perpetuates itself by sparking our desire to *control it all!* Yet, must we allow a theory to predetermine our lives? Is it possible that another method exists that can free us from thinking of ourselves as victims, powerless to deal with our heredity? A different perspective takes into account our genealogy as well as our genes.

## PSYCHOGENETICS: THE BIOLOGY OF BELIEF

Genes refer to single hereditary units that occupy specific locations on a chromosome and determine particular characteristics in an organism. Genealogy denotes ancestry—an entire collection of items and issues within a whole family. This is the family lineage, a composite story of the relationships, culture, education, errors, and fortunes of all family members, imprinted on body and mind through the generations—a genealogical inheritance that we can perpetuate or disown. Genes and genealogy weave themselves together so closely that their connections are invisible. Yet, while genetics is purely scientific, genealogy is our living history, an embodiment of our nature and spirit.

When we examine the family tree from the mindbody perspective, we can pinpoint the errors that continue from generation to generation. Interestingly, though even the thought of an error often provokes feelings of shame and guilt, the true meaning of the word *error* is free of such connotations. The *American Heritage Dictionary* defines *error* as a belief that unintentionally deviates from what is correct, right, or true; its Latin root means "to wander," while the Old Norse root means "to rush." Stop for a moment. Consider if there is anyone you know who does not hold an incorrect belief, who does not wander somehow in thought or action or rush ahead. Surely, it is rare to meet such a person. And certainly, in every family, there is the generational story and the symptom, the familial error and the result.

For example, a girl grows up in a home where her father constantly works. Her mother manages the children and has no time to fulfill her own ambition or to be with her husband. Her resentment seethes; not coincidentally, she suffers from high blood pressure. The girl marries a successful man who also devotes much of his time to work. She feels neglected, represses her anger, and gets pregnant to make her life meaningful. Her obstetrician diagnoses her with hypertension. While conventional medicine would be likely to blame it on the genetic predisposition and cite the pregnancy as the trigger, we don't need a medical background to trace the psychogenetic error.[8] First we can acknowledge the connection between her high blood pressure and her repressed anger through Focusing; then we can Undo the family error of repressed resentment, which leaves us free to Now Act to create a change. The following imagery and drawing exercise is one way to do this. This exercise is for the entire family. All who are interested may participate. It's FUN to do this together and share whatever you discover.

## THE FAMILY TREE

*Intention:* To see and correct the psychogenetic errors.

*Frequency:* Use for 21 days. Take seven days off. Then do for three more cycles.

Close your eyes and breathe out three times. See that you are standing in front of a tree. Know that this is your Family Tree. What does this Family Tree look like? Is it gnarled and stunted or sturdy and tall? Is the foliage abundant or sparse? Are its roots vibrant and embedded firmly in the earth, or are they shallow and withered? How is the trunk? Thick or slim, bent or straight? See if there is any part of the tree that's unhealthy. Breathe out one time. Then in any way that you like, change this image to create a healthier Family Tree that may now bear new fruit (flowers, foliage, healthier roots, and so forth). Once you have done this, breathe out and open your eyes.

After you complete the imagery, fold a page vertically in your notebook. In the left column, draw your experience of the old tree and on the right side draw the new image. Refer to the corrected image daily, without commentary or judgment.

## Using Psychogenetics to Heal Our Children

Our power and will are sapped when we become mesmerized and enslaved by the belief in genetic risk. However, by shifting our focus to psychogenetics, we return to our inherent wisdom. Psychogenetics examines the family belief system and the family errors handed down through the generations, then does whatever is necessary to change them. These errors include long-held resentments, blame, abuse, guilt, addictions, and so forth. Such behaviors influence everything that goes on in the body, for better or worse.

For instance, if both you and your mother have asthma, you need not tell yourself a story about passing the disease on to your child. Instead, you identify the belief system that is repeating itself. Then you make changes in your thinking and behavior that can correct the defective belief gene even *before* your child is born. You may also do this after the fact. That is, you can help your children even if they already have symptoms or are predisposed to asthma. This work is done psychogenetically by changing the belief that lies at the heart of the problem. Do not be surprised when the Skeptic screams "Impossible!" Change is the committee's undoing; it hates when the status quo is threatened. Quite simply, you use the FUN program to create the psychogenetic shift by taking these steps:

- *Focus* by turning toward the difficulty, physical or mental, and looking for the family belief that creates that difficulty.
- *Undo* that belief via work in the invisible world.
- *Now Act* by making corrections to reverse the psychogenetic habits and patterns in everyday life.

## BREAKING FREE OF THE ASTHMATIC IDENTITY

Identifying with family belief systems, stories, myths, and diseases is a custom in our society. Blaming parents is a habit we acquire early on. "You made me do it" and "It's all your fault" are familiar childhood expressions. If children are allowed to believe that asthma is part of their genetic makeup and there's nothing they can do about it, this habitual thought begins to determine their attitudes and actions even beyond asthma. But we can help them break this habit. We do this whenever we encourage them to take responsibility for their feelings and beliefs; when we show them that action has power and value; when we discourage whining, complaining, and blaming; and when we educate them that imagination is more precious than anything money can buy. In *You Learn by Living*, Eleanor Roosevelt writes:

> The most important things in a child's education are curiosity, interest, *imagination*, and a *sense of the adventure* of life. You will find no courses in which these are taught. . . . They are also the qualities that enable us to continue to grow as human beings to the last day of our life.[9]

Unfortunately, society has deprived children of imagination and a sense of adventure. In fact, children have no real childhood anymore. Inundated with computers, video games, and television, children have lost their innocence. They habitually choose the technological world and the material life over the invisible one without understanding their sacrifice. Neil Postman, chair of New York University's School of Communication, Arts and Sciences and author of *The Disappearance of Childhood*, devotes much attention to the effects that technology has on children. Postman says that the story of technology:

> . . . is without a moral center. It puts in its place efficiency, interest and economic advance. It promises heaven on earth

through the conveniences of technological progress. It casts aside all traditional narratives and symbols that suggest stability and orderliness and tells, instead, of a life of skills, technical expertise and the ecstasy of consumption.[10]

Children raised in modern society easily fall prey to this worldview. They neglect nature, their imaginations, and creativity while being consumed with digital wonders. Once they fall into *dis-order*, the asthma arrives to remind us of what has been lost along the way.

As parents, we must take care that we don't abandon the invisible reality and forget our blueprint. When we do, we pass along a dim view to our children, making wonder and wisdom seem extraneous. If we, ourselves, substitute the concrete for the invisible, we can hardly expect our kids to understand that the next material thing or achievement is not all there is. Like adults, children may have little or no idea of who they are, but they are hell-bent on getting what they want. Freedom, however, is not devoid of limits. Before children can heal themselves and become free, they must become responsible. Limits and responsibility are integral to their overall well-being. They help them to mature. When parents make a habit of acquiescing to their children's demands (sweets before dinner, violent television shows, open-ended bedtimes), they create a mutual truce and comfort zone, but they forgo their opportunity to set an example of responsibility and empowerment. For it is only within specified parameters that we experience true freedom.[11]

## LOVE IS A RESPIRATORY EXPERIENCE

But where does love fit in with all this? How do we as parents nurture and love an asthmatic child, or a child with *any* illness, while teaching responsibility and setting boundaries? Just as important, how do we maintain our own health and identity in the midst of the complexities of these day-to-day difficulties? In the 1997 film *As Good as It Gets,* Helen Hunt won an Academy Award for her role as the single mother of an asthmatic son, whom she makes the center of her life and the greater part of her identity. When, through the course of the movie, he improves, she feels lost and bereft rather than joyous. Who is she if she is not the self-sacrificing mother who dedicates her life to her son's asthma? To answer this question, she must redefine her relationship with her child and learn that *Love is a respiratory experience.*[12] Inhalation is analogous to coming together, exhalation to moving apart. Coming together creates a mutual union. Moving apart provides the separation and the space of freedom. She must learn to exhale and let go as well as inhale and draw closer. Without this space we lack the room to breathe.

The following stories about Erica, Emily, Steven, and Kim reveal important information about some of the difficulties involving love and relationship faced by asthmatic children.

## A Teenager's Dilemma

Erica, a thirteen-year-old asthmatic, has just begun to use the FUN program. In one of our meetings, Erica's mother sits beside her. She continually interrupts, answering every question, as though her daughter has lost the capacity to speak for herself. Mom assumes that she is the expert and barely acknowledges her teenaged daughter as a separate person. Erica expresses excitement about going to summer camp. Then, casting a glance at her mom, she adds, "I can't wait to get away from *her.*" Immediately, Mom goes on defensive alert. She warns Erica that at camp she will have to handle the asthma herself. She asks how an inexperienced thirteen-year-old can understand the seriousness of this illness, and she questions how imagery can replace Erica's medication. This is "smother love" in action.

Protectiveness is a natural part of mothering. Mothers are concerned about their kids, even more so when they have asthma. But Erica's mom has gone overboard, dragging her daughter down into her personal quagmire of doubt and fear. However, blaming this parent for her daughter's condition is unfair and unproductive. In fact, we encourage that children *honor* their parents. This makes Erica's remark about getting "away from *her*" inappropriate and unhealthy. *Now* is the moment for Mom to set some boundaries, to put her foot down. Honor, respect, good manners—qualities that seem threatened with extinction in our society—do not imply repression. They demonstrate moderation, self-respect, and responsibility. Erica is out of order when she speaks disparagingly of her mother. Lost boundaries and compromised identities present some of the most difficult issues for asthmatic children and their parents to resolve.

From a mindbody perspective, Erica's symptoms emerge as the result of two opposing wishes. She feels bound to the image of herself as her mother sees her, and at the same time she wants to break free. She's torn apart by her need to stay connected with this parent (especially since her father is unavailable), and her natural adolescent desire to become her own person. Meanwhile, this mother's protective instincts blind her to her daughter's dilemma. She who wants "nothing but the best" for her child unwittingly creates an impasse. Erica feels angry about the limitations imposed by her mother but lacks the means to express it. Her anger exacerbates the asthma, which becomes the mutual identity of mother and child. They become entrapped and entwined; accordingly, the disease makes its statement. To heal this relationship, they must separate and create a space of freedom. Camp is a wonderful way to begin an *Undoing* of their old habits.

### Emily and Sara: A Story of Hope and Healing

Emily is nine. Since a week after Emily's birth, her mom, Sara, had been going through surgeries for borderline ovarian tumor. Often Sara could not be with her daughter because of her illness. At three, Emily developed asthma. At the same time, Sara was diagnosed with ovarian cancer. Sara's own words best describe this situation and its resolution:

We enjoyed our lives with the sweetness of discovery a young child brings to it, yet there was always an underlying current of fear. Just as I had been scheduled to reenter the hospital for another surgery, Emily began coughing every twelve seconds and could not stop. I realized how the coughing was linked to our emotional upset. Emily's coughing was finally brought under control with Prednisone and the use of a nebulizer; but for me, the diagnosis this time was ovarian cancer. I began chemotherapy. Though successful at first, when the therapy was done the numbers slowly crept back up.

I knew that there was nothing more that standard medicine could do for me. I was not willing to abuse my immune system further, and I wanted to get to the bottom of the recurrences. Soon after this decision, I began to do imagery work. Within three months the markers were at nearly normal levels. I then introduced this work to Emily, who healed herself of the asthma within seven days. [Emily tells her story later on.] I started to learn about living life in the present, and the calm and peace brought a joy to our household that liberated us from the fear that had previously dominated our lives.

This young child was deeply affected by her mother's illness. Her body had absorbed the grief she and her parent experienced, and it manifested in her lungs. Looking at love as a "respiratory experience," we see that Emily and Sara's natural process of coming together and moving apart—in other words, their life's breath—was threatened by cancer. The rhythm of their mutual union collapsed. Emily wanted and needed to be with her mother without the threat of losing her, and so she held on for dear life. There was no middle ground, no safe way to release her breath and create a space. Though Emily's situation seems the reverse of Erica's where "over-parenting" was the issue, the result was the same. The delicate life-love balance had been compromised. And Emily's asthma presented itself.

Sara knew her daughter's health crisis had passed when one day, as she was saying good-bye to Emily, her daughter kissed her on the lips. "I realized at that moment that she was no longer afraid of losing me, that now she believed I was well and she could finally allow herself to love me."

Sara's encounter with serious illness marked a turning point in the lives of the family. No longer could they take anything for granted. Each day, each breath was precious. Sara's survival and healing from cancer created a new relationship with Emily.

In her own words, nine-year old Emily describes her experience:

Before I did imagery, ever since I was two I was on medication every day for four years. I was on allergy medications from two years old to three years old, and on asthma medication from three years old to six. Once I had been doing imagery for one week we went back to the doctor to tell him that it was gone. He told us, "It will be back in the fall when the allergy season starts." I now only go to the doctor for school checkups.

When I went into my body to see what was making my asthma, I saw something that looked like a "Sun" and something that looked like a "Moon." The "Sun" and the "Moon" were fighting. I helped the Sun win and so the Sun won and the Moon lost. Then I saw that there was a rainbow over the Sun and a devil over the Moon. The Moon left and he only comes back when I have a stomachache. Now that I don't have the Moon anymore I don't have any more asthma. I kept doing imagery to keep the asthma out, and I still do it sometimes when I get a stomachache or when something is bothering me.[13]

Note: The imagery exercise that Emily used was "The Exorcism" from chapter 7.

Since her first imagery experience, Emily has not used conventional medication. When she senses a breathing problem coming

on, her treatment of choice is imagination. Often, she uses imagery
spontaneously, making up exercises as she goes along, then writing
and drawing what she sees. She reports that now the sun *and* the
moon are willing to help her. For extra healing power, she brings in
the stars and places them in her lungs, too. The benefits Emily reaps
from this work extend beyond symptomatic relief. When she reports
seeing angels in her room, no one laughs or tries to convince her
they're not real. Imagination is valued. The invisible world is discussed and revered. Looking at life this way is a family affair, one
that cultivates and sustains this precious union of mother and child.

## School Daze

Barbara and her six-year-old son Steven found first grade a traumatic experience. Barbara woke in the morning and used all her
energy just to get Steven dressed, as he ran through the house and
hid from her. When they finally arrived at school, he would throw
himself on the floor of the classroom and scream. He made it perfectly clear how much he hated it.

From the time Kim was in third grade, she woke up each morning and demanded that her parents check to see if "it" had burned
down yet. Kim was talking about her school. She couldn't stand
going, though her parents didn't know why.

Steven and Kim are asthmatics. They also hate school and don't
hesitate to show it. Undoubtedly, they dislike having asthma. Yet if
an attack means staying home, that makes the asthma a lot more tol-
erable. This does not mean that they consciously make themselves
sick. Yet it does bring up an important example of the kind of pressures our children suffer in their daily lives and the way they respond.

But why, you might ask, should school present any more of a
problem now than it has in the past? And what does it have to do
with relationship and love? In an important way, school is also a
respiratory experience. Our children's identities and lives are
defined by it more than ever before. Kids today feel greater pressure
to perform. Fierce competition begins in kindergarten. Parents

worry whether Johnny will get into the Ivy League even before he can write his name, whether nine-year-old Jane will be a doctor like her mother.

At a kids' tree-trimming contest in an affluent New York suburb, the same third grade moms who pushed to have their children accepted into a gifted-child program stood guard and directed their kids' every move. They seemed to care far more about their child winning first place than their having FUN. This type of pressure can be stifling; it raises fears and suppresses freedom. It does not foster ease and mutuality in the parent-child relationship. With additional activities like music, organized sports, religious training, and special preparatory tutoring, children have little if any separation from pressured activities, no space for plain old FUN. Some families don't mind, or at least they don't complain—certain kids even thrive on their busy schedules—but many feel pressed, put upon, edgy. Often, they hardly have time to take a breath.

For children with a tendency toward asthma, this academic pressure cooker can be disastrous. It certainly does not strengthen their value systems or improve their sense of themselves. Of course, as parents we want our children to do well. But does doing well mean the same thing to them as it does to us? Imposing such serious limitations on our children's freedom, even though we're sure it's in their best interests, comes at a price that we may not be willing to pay. If we want our children to breathe freely, doesn't it make sense to help them enjoy their childhood before they plunge headfirst into the whirlpool that we call adult life?

Our children are much more than our future. They are our *present*. Their asthmatic condition tells us about society's condition as well as their own. Conventional drugs and research eliminate symptoms, whereas an education in responsibility and awareness addresses the illness and all it implies. The best medicine is one that affects the heart and the mind as well as the bronchial tubes and the lungs. A mindbody education teaches that thoughts, words, and actions resonate in the world; kindness to others and to ourselves can heal; we are valuable and lovable just as we are; and errors can be learning tools. This gives children the room they need for learning, and for breathing freely.

## NOW THAT WE KNOW

Psychogenetics, the respiratory quality of love, the healing power of humor, and the importance of taking responsibility are more than just interesting concepts. They are the DNA of self-empowerment for our children. By integrating these concepts into our own lives, we can pass them along through example. Thus they can learn to live without fear of the next attack, and they can release their attachment to asthma as an identity or an excuse.

Since kids are natural FUNsters, we have created a FUN chapter just for them where we introduce them to the FUN approach. This includes imagery and several other techniques. We suggest they do as much as they can on their own and that you make yourself available for questions or reports on their progress. Provide them with a special notebook in which to do this work and the space in which to explore this themselves. Resist the temptation to give unbidden advice. Some kids take to this process more easily than others. Allow them to come to it in their own way, at their own pace. Even if they do just one exercise, it can be of tremendous value.

Introducing your children to this program through the FUN Guide does more than address the asthma. You teach them to appreciate the inner life, and they learn that illness need not be a life sentence. Many of the exercises throughout this book can serve your children well. Give them credit for their ability to learn, to be flexible, to follow a different path than the one they have been on until now. Instead of seeing the asthma as the monster out to get them, allow it to be an opportunity for change, for growth, and for a beautiful unfolding into a free, productive, and happy life.

### CHAPTER 10

# THE FUN GUIDE FOR KIDS

*Throw off the bowlines. Sail away from the safe harbor.*
*Catch the trade winds in your sails. Explore. Dream.*
*Discover.*

MARK TWAIN

<table>
<tr><td>

**THE CONTENTS**

- What is the FUN Guide?
- Imagine Being Well
- Your Favorite Things
- The FUN Collage

</td></tr>
</table>

## WHAT IS THE FUN GUIDE?

The FUN Guide is a special chapter just for kids. Having FUN is an important part of life. Here in the FUN Guide, you will find some exercises to help you do that. They can also help you feel healthier. When you have an asthma symptom, these exercises will give you a new kind of medicine to use. This kind of medicine is different from the kind you usually take. It's called Mind Medicine. We call it that because it shows you how to use your mind in a new way—a way that can make you feel healthy, happy, and strong. If there is anything you do not understand or can't do on your own, just ask someone for help.

## IMAGINE BEING WELL

Your imagination is a very special thing. And you can use it in wonderful ways. Here in the FUN Guide, you will find something we call *Imagery*. When you use imagery, you see things from the *inside* instead of from the outside—something like the way you do when you dream. There are instructions at the beginning of chapter 4 on what to do before you image. Read these before you begin. Then choose the exercises you want to use and see what happens. Don't overdo by trying them all at once. Decide which ones you like best, and make them a part of your FUN Plan for Healing.

---

### THE PINE FOREST[1]✴

*When to use:* The next time you feel an asthma symptom starting up.
   *How often:* At the beginning of an attack for two to three minutes.
   Close your eyes. Breathe out three times and see yourself in a forest filled with tall, fragrant pine trees. Stand next to one of these trees, and breathe in its clear piney smell. As you breathe out, imagine the air going all the way down through your body and out through the bottoms of your feet. See this air coming out as gray smoke and being buried deep in the earth. Do this a few times— breathe in the piney smell, breathe out the old, stale air. Then open your eyes, knowing you are now breathing easily.

---

### THE RAINBOW BRIDGE ✴

*When to use:* To breathe freely. To get rid of any asthma symptoms.
   *How often:* Use whenever you have a symptom. Or once a day for 21 days.

Close your eyes and breathe out three times. See a rainbow in the sky above you. Begin to walk across it to the other side. As you go across, feel its beautiful colors moving through you. Imagine these rainbow colors going right into your lungs and filling them with light. When you get across, know that you have left all the symptoms behind. Feel how you are now breathing freely and easily. See what you find there on the other side. Then open your eyes.

## THE BUBBLE HELMET *

*When to use:* When you need protection from bad air.

*How often:* Whenever you are in a place where the air is bad for you, use this exercise as much and as often as you need it.

Close your eyes. Imagine you are wearing a round, clear, bubble helmet on your head. See that where you breathe in through the helmet, there is a fine gold screen that filters out all the bad air. See the air coming in as blue light. Know that only good, pure air can enter your lungs when you are wearing this helmet. When you are ready, open your eyes and continue whatever you are doing, while knowing the helmet is still in place.

## More Imagery Exercises

Here, we have listed the names of three more imagery exercises that are found in other sections of the book.

- *The Exorcism:* Emily, who tells how she healed herself from asthma in chapter 9, began with this exercise. You'll find it in chapter 7.
- *The Golden Inhaler:* Use this exercise from chapter 4 whenever you would usually use your regular inhaler.

- *Box of Balloons:* Helen used this to get rid of asthma, to feel light and free, in chapter 9.

*Just for Fun:* Write or draw what you see and what happens in the imagery. Do this in the special notebook you use for this work.

## MY FAVORITE THINGS:
## CREATE YOUR OWN IMAGERY

Making up your own imagery can be a FUN thing to do. Try this. First, take some time to think about your favorite things. What are your favorite places, toys, games, colors, and stories? What are the things you like to do best (sports, dancing, singing, swimming)? Make a list of these in your notebook. If you need help, ask for it. You may work on this for a few minutes or for a few days. Add new favorite things as you go along.

Now choose something from this list that you want to use for an imagery exercise. Earlier, Emily used the image of the sun and the moon fighting inside her lungs. This came from a story she had read. Here is an example of how to make up imagery with one of your favorite things: Jeffrey has a toy sailboat he loves. He sometimes takes it to the park and sails it on the pond. He gets a good feeling as he sets the boat free to skim across the calm water, pushed by the wind. Jeffrey also loves to go out in a full-sized sailboat on breezy summer days. He uses this exercise whenever the asthma begins to bother him. Jeffrey closes his eyes, and this is what he imagines:

## THE SAILBOAT ✹

I see myself sailing my toy boat at the park. It moves across the water, and I see the sails puffing out. At the same time I feel my chest filling with clean fresh air just like the sails. Then I imagine that I am on the boat. Suddenly the wind picks us up, and we go floating off into the sky. I look down and I laugh. I am on a flying boat, high in the sky, and I am free. Everything on the ground looks very small. When I come back down, my chest feels open and my breathing is fine.

Amanda loves *The Wizard of Oz*, so she created the next exercise. She uses it whenever her chest feels like it is getting tight or heavy.

## MELTING THE WITCH ✹

I see myself all dressed up as a Good Witch. I go inside my lungs and see there the Bad Witch, who is squeezing my chest. I wave my magic wand and cast a spell on the Bad Asthma Witch, who immediately melts (just like the one in *The Wizard of Oz*). When the Bad Witch is all melted, the wheezing disappears.

You can make up your own imagery just like Amanda and Jeffrey. There is no right or wrong way to do this. Whatever you choose to do is fine. Just try it and see what happens. Write down the exercises you make up in your notebook. Use them whenever you like.

## THE FUN COLLAGE

How would you look, feel, play, and live without the asthma in your life? Did you ever hear the saying "seeing is believing"? The FUN Collage helps you to see how it would be to live asthma free. You can also make a FUN collage as a family project.

---

### MAKING A FUN COLLAGE

- Find pictures of yourself smiling, looking healthy and happy, by yourself and with people you love. Also find other little things like shells from the beach or tickets to a ball game or to a funny movie—anything at all that gives you pleasure.
- Put these together on a large piece of cardboard or heavy paper in a way that you like.
- Paste or tape them on so they won't fall off.
- Hang this where it can remind you of the way that you want to be—healthy, happy, living asthma free!
- Change this at any time. Add other things you find as you go along. Get rid of anything you no longer want or need.
- Look at this every day and smile three times.

---

You have come to the end of the FUN Guide. But there is always more you can do to heal the asthma and keep having fun. Add new ideas to your list of Favorite Things. Make up your own exercises. Ask your parents about other exercises in this book that you might try. Remember, there is no right or wrong way to do this. Just as long as you have FUN!

In chapter 12 you will find a special kids' plan for living asthma free.

### CHAPTER 11

# THE
# MINDBODY WAY

## Environment, Nutrition,
## and Exercise-Induced Asthma

*Being willing to change allows you to move from one
point of view to a viewing point—a higher, more expan-
sive place where you can see both sides.*

THOMAS CRUM

This chapter is the natural outgrowth of all that has gone before.
It offers practical techniques to address the three major areas identified by conventional medicine as powerful triggers for asthma.
While you read this, we ask that you separate yourself, at least temporarily, from your beliefs regarding the various *causes* of asthma—
environmental allergies, food products, exercise—and open
yourself, instead, to an experience of wholeness, connection, and
meaning.

Although people ordinarily separate one type of asthma from
another, we propose instead that "asthma is asthma." Thus, despite
variations in symptoms or triggers, the issue that lies beneath the
surface is the same. This issue is *freedom*—freedom from smothering relationships, freedom to be oneself, freedom to choose, and

freedom to enjoy and experience life. This chapter helps you cultivate these freedoms through perceptions and processes that allow
you to release attachments—to beliefs, feelings, attitudes, possessions, and even to your breath. Though it must seem strange to
hear that your attachment to breathing precludes your freedom,
remind yourself that life begins on the exhale. It is, indeed, your
letting go, especially of your breath, that generates freedom.

To become your own authority is the key. Experts don't have
all the answers. What they advise may work well for others but may
not work as well for you. The same medication, diet, and prevention techniques can't be trusted to deliver the same results: notice
that there's always some new, improved remedy, diet, theory, or
method being touted as the latest miracle cure. Only when you
look *within*, to the emotional, social, and spiritual issues at asthma's
core, can you truly begin to heal. The next story illustrates how
this works.

## THE BREAKTHROUGH

Julia had her first asthma symptoms when she was five. Her attacks
sometimes were so serious she required emergency treatment at the
hospital. By seven, her parents had taken her for allergy testing at
Children's Hospital in Boston. Here they were told that Julia's
asthma was caused by her allergy to feathers—to the down pillows
she slept on, the down sofa she sat on, the down quilt on her bed.
According to Julia, it took her thirty years to understand that it
wasn't the feathers but something within herself that lay at the root
of her problem.

Julia's healing came about through a sudden shift in her perception of an ongoing family situation that had dominated her life
since the beginning. Julia's older brother died in a car accident
when he was twenty. From her earliest memories he had always
been in trouble—at home, in school, with the police. By five, Julia

knew that her parents had their hands full, that the best she could do in that volatile situation was to make no waves. She virtually held her breath trying not to be a bother.

Two years ago, Julia and her partner, Deb, a physician with a deep interest in mindbody work, visited Julia's hometown, where they spent an evening with an old and dear friend of her parents. Over dinner they reminisced about the atmosphere Julia grew up in—how difficult her brother was and what a hard time her parents had gone through with him. Later that evening, Deb spoke the words that shone a light into the darkness of Julia's past: "It must have been tough being in that volatile environment with such con-flict between your parents and brother," she said. "You must have been so tense you could hardly breathe."

"Yes. It *was* tough to breathe in that situation," Julia said. "But now is not then. That's all in the past." As she spoke these words aloud, suddenly the origin of the asthma became clear. In that instant she knew she no longer needed this disease in her body, and she was finally able to release it. That night, for the first time since she was seven, Julia slept on a feather bed with a down pillow and has been doing so ever since. She admits to keeping an inhaler in her medicine cabinet, just in case. But since her direct experience of this shift in her thinking and physiology, she knows that her mind is much more powerful than that inhaler. Julia says she now carries with her, at every moment, the most powerful medication of all—an ability to be aware of and in touch with this mindbody connection. For her, this alone has created a healing. The feathers no longer present an issue. Saying the words aloud, recognizing there was another option besides being sick, was the final step in letting go of the past and becoming free.

Julia's experience notwithstanding, asthmatic or allergic responses to certain irritants do exist. Smoke exacerbates asthma. Cat fur provokes allergic reactions. Dairy products produce mucus, which in turn clogs the lungs. The point, however, as was brought so clearly to life in the previous story, is that your reaction relates not just to the irritant but to your whole being. The stimulus is not the *reason* for the illness, it simply adds to what *already* exists, enfolded in your consciousness. Thus, when you separate mental, emotional, spiritual, and physical issues and designate one as The Cause, healing becomes impossible.

With this in mind, we offer you a mindbody overview of concerns that asthmatics have regarding environment, nutrition, and exercise. Using a mindbody perspective, you go beyond the common approach to these issues. We propose that as you consider this information, you become your own authority: keep only what resonates for you and "let go" of the rest.

## EMISSARIES OF THE ENVIRONMENT

Environmentally related asthma tests our control. And what a test it is! We try to control our contact with, and reaction to dust, dust mites, pollens, molds, and toxic fumes. Nevertheless, when we see the environment only in terms of the physical reality, we leave out a big piece of the picture. Your true environment is a state of being—your internal climate, composed of what goes on within yourself as well as what happens out there. Your thoughts, your feelings, your responses to family, friends, work, and play are all environmental issues. And you can no more isolate these elements than you can separate inhalation from exhalation or breath from life.

Noxious thoughts are as damaging to your health as toxic fumes; they lurk unseen and show up as emotional and physical symptoms. Discord at work harms your lungs; it prevents you from breathing deeply and exhaling fully. Discontent and anger molder away in your mind and create bodily reactions as surely as the mold in your basement. They nurture themselves on the darkness of thought that eventually embeds itself in your heart. When you approach your environment with an awareness such as this, born of genuine meaning, you gain dominion over a part of your life that usually seems beyond your control.

Julia, whose asthma was diagnosed as a reaction to feathers in her home environment, lived a profoundly circumscribed life, one that she cocreated with her family. Ordinarily, Julia could not permit herself to be "an issue" for her parents. But when the feathers triggered the asthma, that made it okay to get some attention. The asthma held several meanings and served multiple purposes, all invisible to the unreceptive eye. It was also a glyph for the loss and anger she felt. But the feathers were not the cause. When Julia realized this, she opened the door to a new way of thinking and a new way of living her life.

The FUN method enables you to see your physical reactions as messages and involves the following three steps:

- Focus on the inner environment as well as the outer one.
- Undo the toxic beliefs and sayings of the Committee that poison your body and mind.
- Now Act, in ways that bring this inner shift out into the world.

On a practical level, a thorough cleanup of your environment can be complex and expensive. However, we have two suggestions for detoxifying your emotional environment and, in turn, altering your physical one. The first is both a Focusing and Undoing process in which you use imagination to clean a room in your home from top to bottom. With the second, you physically clean out old stuff. Both encourage the understanding that to clean your emotional environment is to clean yourself.

## CLEANING THE ROOM [1]

*Intention:* To clean yourself emotionally and mentally. To use as a preventive technique.

*Frequency:* Use once. Then use thereafter as desired.

Close your eyes and breathe out three times. Imagine a significant room in your home. Move all the furniture (in your imagination) to the center of the room. Take down the pictures and draperies and bring them to the center of the room. Put them on the bed, if it is in the center, or in a container. Now discard whatever you do not want. Bring in the necessary cleaning tools, including a ladder. Begin with the ceiling and thoroughly clean the room from top to bottom, including the windows, walls, and floors. If anything needs to be polished, including floors and furniture, do this too. When you are finished, put back whatever you want to keep. Place the rest in containers or bags, take it outside, and burn it or sink it in water, with weights attached, until it disappears to the bottom. Focus on the feelings and thoughts you experience while the discarded items burn (or sink to the bottom of a lake or the ocean). Then return to the room, go inside, and see how you feel and what you notice. Keep anything healthy or good that you discover for yourself. Then breathe out and open your eyes.

Often a brief version of this exercise can provide immediate help when a symptom threatens. Emily, the child in chapter 9 who created a truce between the sun and the moon, spontaneously created a simplified version of this. One morning, as she felt a symptom coming on, she told her mom that she needed to clean her room. Then she remarked that the room she needed to clean was not the one upstairs in their house but the one upstairs in her head. Once she did the imagery, the symptom vanished.

After you complete this imaginal room cleaning, fold a page in your notebook vertically in half. Write your experience on the left and draw your images on the right, then sign your name. This exercise may indicate certain actions, such as painting a room in a particular color, bringing in flowers and plants, hanging a picture, or getting rid of things. Following through on what needs to be changed is the path to action. The next exercise is the physical counterpart of the preceding one.

## RELEASING OLD STUFF

*Intention:* To remove negative influences and physical clutter.

*Frequency:* Do for seven days. Then continue for two more weeks if necessary.

*Physically* clean out old stuff from the past and get rid of it (clothes, mementos, letters, papers, and so forth). As you do this, know that you are releasing what you do not need in your life and creating a free space in your head, your heart, and your lungs. Continue to do this for as long as it takes to remove the old, unclean influences.

## To Summarize

The feathers, the mold, the dander, the dust—all actually can be irritants. We do not suggest that you disregard these physical triggers but rather that you do not dwell on them and blame them for your symptoms. Relate first to the nature of the allergen itself. Then, when the symptom occurs, ask yourself, Who am I with? Where am I? What's going on? How do I feel? Dust, mold, pollens, animals, and toxins are coded clues, not causes. They indicate a sensitivity and refer you to the core situation by way of the asthmatic symptom.

## NUTRITION: WHAT IS IT ABOUT FOOD?

Second only to our resistance to changing our minds is our reluctance to change our diets. If it's true that "with our thoughts we create the world" and "we are what we eat," no wonder we are in such a fix. When we fail to realize the importance and intimacy of our relationship with food, we trivialize an area of life basic to existence. Our everyday language overflows with food imagery. We say, "Something is eating me"; "sweet as apple pie"; "the deal went sour"; "thick as molasses"; "cool as a cucumber"; "food for thought." It's not unusual for us to call our loved ones "Sweetie Pie," "Pumpkin," "Cookie," "Honey," "Pork Chop," "Lamb Chop," "Lamby Pie," and "Sweet Cakes." Ignoring the symptoms of our bodies' discontent, we eat even what doesn't agree with us, ingesting an array of antacid medications that tell our stomachs, in no uncertain terms, to shut up.

Food is a loaded issue. Conventional nutritionists give us lists of dos and don'ts, yet they fail to explain that our individual beliefs as well as our digestive systems determine our reactions. For instance: people with dissociative identity disorder,[2] more commonly known as multiple personality, may have an allergic reaction in one personality while not in another. For example, the Mary persona may be allergic to milk products, while the Marcia persona can drink as much milk as she likes.[3] When Mary makes a mental shift so that her beliefs, attitudes, and feelings become those of Marcia, her biology and brain/body chemistry transform as well. This strange and true phenomenon demonstrates just how powerful the mind really is and further illuminates the process involved in Julia's spontaneous healing.

A less startling example involves Rebecca, a client with a "delicate stomach." Fried foods, hot dogs and hamburgers, anything greasy, too cold, too rich, or too sweet gives Rebecca severe indigestion—except when she is with a certain friend. With this person, Rebecca can eat anything! No reflux, no cramps, just FUN. Rebecca believes the laughter and enjoyment she experiences with this person (who never has a problem with food) enable her to shift into what she calls her Superwoman mode—an image of digestive impunity. She assumes a persona and a belief that diminish her food sensitivities along with her concerns about the future and the past. This experience is exquisite proof of the physical changes generated by our beliefs and thoughts.

## Knowing What's Right for You

If you are a square peg, you can't squeeze yourself into a round hole; it won't work no matter how hard you try. To determine your nutritional plan based only on your being part of the population labeled asthmatic undermines your ability to choose. Self-knowledge is the key to judicious decision making. Before you run to others, who supposedly know more than you, consult your dreams, imagination, intuition, and the glyphs of your daily life. These are your connections to your wisest self. They refer you to your blueprint and allow you to make sense of what's going on.

## Personal Dream Medicine

Nancy had suffered from intestinal pain and nausea that woke her during the night, caused her pain immediately after eating, and had plagued her for almost two weeks. The doctor she consulted advised a strong antacid medication and a battery of invasive tests. But Nancy felt uncomfortable about following advice that she sensed was overzealous and in her case inappropriate. Instead, she chose to ask her dreams how she might heal herself. The next night, she dreamed that she met two elderly women who stood before a large crystal bowl filled with blackberries. She asked their permission, then filled a small bowl with some berries, said thank-you, and went on her way. When Nancy awoke, she understood that the dream held the healing remedy she had sought. That same day, she began eating blackberries. Almost immediately she felt their effect. Within a week the symptoms faded to practically nothing. She then continued with her dream remedy for about six months, until she was completely healed.

Later, an herbalist explained to Nancy that, yes, blackberries were a healing remedy, effective for soothing inflammation in the intestines. Somehow, her dream reflected her intuitive knowledge of this natural medicine. In addition to eating the blackberries, Nancy, who had been using the FUN program, asked herself: "What am I inflamed about?" "What am I burning to do?" "What belief has made me seek out a steady diet of rich foods?"

By listening to her dream, she received a healing remedy. By listening to her body, she recognized her desire for a richer life— one that required sacrifices she had been unwilling to make until her difficulty arose. Eating fatty, heavy foods had been Nancy's way of creating this life, but her body would no longer cooperate. This required her to change the food she fed her *mind* as well as the food she fed her body. She had to let go of the pastries, the cheese, the chocolate. The sacrifice was necessary if she wanted to move forward. Nancy made the corrections, repaired the damage, and took another step toward becoming her own authority.

With this perspective and these techniques, you can find out what's right for you, whether that's acupuncture, herbs, dreams, imagination, or a more conventional approach. If the Skeptic complains that this story is not about an asthma symptom, he's missing the point. *All inflammatory processes,* whether connected to asthma, intestinal issues, or allergic reactions, are related. In mindbody medicine, a remedy you create from imagination or discover in dreams may apply to more than one physical or emotional symptom. You too can follow Nancy's example and consult the wisdom of your dreams. Be direct. Ask which foods heal and which foods harm. You may be surprised by the answers.

## THE DILEMMA OF EXERCISE-INDUCED ASTHMA

Mark works as a financial consultant on Wall Street. Success drives him, not only at work, but in everything he does. For years his morning run has been important to him. But recently, instead of feeling energized, he feels depleted. His chest gets tight, his shoulders feel heavy, he finds it harder to breathe, and he is forced to slow his pace. Immediately afterward, Mark starts coughing and wheezing, particularly in cold weather. When his doctor diagnosed him with exercise-induced asthma, Mark was devastated. He wondered how this could happen and why to him.

Exercise-induced asthma, commonly known as EIA, is particularly frustrating. Those who have it are active, invested in their bodies, interested in getting in shape and staying that way. Often they are accomplished and bright. Yet their lungs betray them; every time they run or exercise strenuously they risk an attack. While many conventional sources provide practical ways to prevent and relieve EIA, they concentrate only on the physical mechanics. What's missing, however, is the mindbody perspective.

The fact that the asthma is induced by exercise implies something more than its connection to physical exertion. Once again, we suggest you turn toward the difficulty, in this case, the "exercise." Pay attention first to the personal meaning and purpose that exercise holds for you. While many sources provide conventional advice on how to stem exercise-induced attacks, here we offer several mindbody techniques for both deeper healing and symptom relief. These include: Healing by Definition, an Etymology Rx, and an EIA Imagery Regimen.

## Healing by Definition

*Webster's Ninth Dictionary* defines exercise as "the act of bringing into play or realizing in action." Stop for a moment, and consider the following questions as though your inner physician were asking them of you during a meditation or a dream. Suspend disbelief. Instead of looking for the instant fix, look within.

Ask yourself:

- What do I want or need to *bring into play?*
- What *action* do I want or need to *realize* in my life?

As you answer each question, write down whatever comes up for you. Another technique is to ask yourself these questions before you go to sleep. Write the question in your imagination or in your notebook. Then ask for a dream that tells you how the symptom defines your life. What is it you need to change or release? When you get an answer, pay attention. There is no deeper, more powerful healing remedy than dream medicine, which as you have seen in this chapter can be translated into a healing remedy in everyday life.

## An Etymology Rx

*Exercitare* means "to drive out." As the Latin etymological root of the word *exercise*, it is particularly intriguing. How extraordinary! By going to the root of the word *exercise*, we arrive, full circle, at the root or core of all the asthma exercises, "The Exorcism." Not coincidentally, this exercise intends to *drive out* the influence of the one, or ones, who interfere with your ability to breathe, who bear down, control, restrict, and become your authority. If Mark, the Wall Street broker we referred to earlier, would stop and consider who or what drives him to attain perfection, even when he runs, he might be able to breathe more easily. Better still, Mark could do "The Exorcism" imagery.

To transform your relationship with exercise, do "The Exorcism," even if you have already done it. Make it your conscious intention to *exorcise* or "drive out" those inside you who are sabotaging your ability to *exercise* freely. Now ask yourself: Who or what do I need to drive out? See what happens, then write and draw it in your notebook.

## The EIA Imagery Regimen

The imagery included here is its own form of exercise—a mental one that affects body, mind, and spirit. It can provide you with renewed vigor and help you break the frustrating and frightening loop of enslavement called EIA. We do not advise that you use these exercises all at once. Instead, start with one or two as a daily practice, and use the immediate symptom relief exercises as needed. In the next chapter we will delineate a special 21-day plan for those with EIA that includes other techniques and practices as well.

The first exercise provides you with a simple way to generate physiological change through imaginal jogging. This is a perfect inner practice to accompany your physical exercise program and can improve its effectiveness.

---

## THE RED SUIT [4]

*Intention:* To run and breathe freely.

*Frequency:* Use before you run or exercise.

Close your eyes. Breathe out three times, and see yourself putting on a red jogging suit and red sneakers. See yourself going out of your house or apartment and walking to the park. Enter the park, and begin to run around it clockwise, becoming aware of everything you see. Become aware of what you sense and feel, of the wind passing by you. Become aware of your stride and your breathing. Notice the trees, grass, and sky. Sense how as you are running, your lungs are functioning perfectly and rhythmically. Complete your run by coming back to the point at which you started. Walk out of the park and back to your home. Take off the jogging clothes, shower, dry off, and put on the clothes you are going to wear for the day. Then breathe out and open your eyes.

---

The following exercises appear in other chapters of the book. We list them here with their intentions. Some will be part of the 21-day plan. Select whichever appeal to you. Try them and see what happens.

## In Chapter 4

- *Golden Inhaler:* To give you a way to reduce or replace the use of your regular inhaler.
- *Golden Bellows:* To strengthen and heal the respiratory system. To increase lung capacity.
- *Taking the Weight off Your Chest:* To alleviate and remove symptoms of asthma.

## In Chapter 7

- *The Exorcism:* To heal the lungs.
- *The Singing Lung:* To Undo or prevent difficulty in breathing. To have FUN!

## In Chapter 8

- *The Triple Mirror:* To generate action and healing.

## THE NEW VIEW

When you look at the issues discussed in this chapter, you might think of them in the following way: your environmental home mirrors the house of your heart; the food that sustains your body nourishes your soul; your movement in life reflects the movement of your spirit. Instead of focusing on your difficulties by looking for causes and reasons, by separating the physical, emotional, moral, and spiritual aspects one from another, look within yourself at your innate wholeness. Focus on your blueprint, see where you may have compromised yourself and gone astray. And begin to live by your own truth. This, more than any antihistamine, nutrition plan, or world-famous expert, will liberate you from your symptoms and enable you to live asthma free.

### CHAPTER 12

# ASTHMA FREE
# IN 21 DAYS

## Your Mindbody Plan for Healing

*Even if you are on the right track, you will get run over if you just sit there.*

WILL ROGERS

At this point, you have read enough. Now it's time for action. To this end we have organized the exercises from the previous chapters into three 21-day healing plans—one for adults, one for those with exercise-induced asthma, and one for children. These plans are suggestions; they are not meant to be rigid or authoritarian. They offer, instead, flexible ways for you to practice what you have read and learned. Be your own authority, take responsibility for your health and wellness, and use the plans you find here for living asthma free, or design your own.

### The Complete Exercise Index

This index lists all the exercises in the book with their intentions, divided by chapter headings, so you can easily locate them. Use the plan of your choice for 21 days. When you're done, you can use the same plan again to continue your healing process, or you can amend it and try something new. Go ahead. Experiment. Have FUN! The index will help remind you of the many choices available to you. Remember, although these plans may be likened to healing prescriptions, they are not "doctors' orders." They are, instead, a way to create a more intimate relationship with your own inner physician.

*Keep These Five Pointers in Mind*

1. Imagery creates the deepest changes when practiced for 21 days. Use those exercises that most appeal to you as well as ones that address uncomfortable issues that remain unresolved.
2. Taking action involves drawing, music, collage, writing, exercise, and other constructive activities for daily life. These offer you a chance to tap into your creative potential.
3. With exercises that ask you questions of self-discovery, write your answers in your notebook and refer to them periodically, to see where you have been and where you are now.
4. We recommend that you use the full plan at least once and then choose the parts you want to continue and those you want to change. You decide.
5. Exercises that are essential to the success of the program are marked with a ✳. Make sure you include these in your practice to ensure the best possible result.

*Note: Before you begin your program, make sure you have filled in the Asthma Questionnaire and the Belief Inventory.*

## THE 21-DAY HEALING PLAN FOR ADULTS

### Week One

- sstuff: Exercise for Panic Prevention—chapter 3
- The Exorcism ✳: A deep healing for your lungs and your life—chapter 7

- The Golden Inhaler ✳: For immediate symptom relief—
  chapter 4
- Draw the Symptom: To define the symptom and bring inside
  to outside—chapter 6
- The Freedom Exercise: To generate freedom and healing—
  chapter 5
- Do unto Yourself: Be kind to yourself, generate joy—
  chapter 8

## Week Two

Continue to use: sstuff, Golden Inhaler, Freedom, Do unto Your-self. Continue The Exorcism if you feel there is more to be accom-plished, for two more weeks. Then, add the following:

- Taking a Weight off Your Chest ✳: To relieve and remove
  symptoms—chapter 4
- Writing to Heal: To eliminate symptoms and need for
  medication—chapter 7
- Create Your Own Top Twenty: Use music to express emotions
  and heal your life—chapter 7
- Turning Things Around: To disempower the Committee—
  chapter 7

## Week Three

Continue to use: sstuff, Inhaler, Freedom, Do unto Yourself, Top Twenty, Turning Things Around. Add the following:

- Two of You: To give unconditional love to yourself—
  chapter 6
- The Triple Mirror: To generate change, growth, and action—
  chapter 8
- Create a Prayer Collage: To begin an asthma-free life—
  chapter 8
- Releasing Old Stuff: Release stuff from your past and free up
  your life—chapter 11

# THE 21-DAY HEALING PLAN FOR
# EXERCISE-INDUCED ASTHMA

## Week One
- ssTUFF: Exercise for Panic Prevention—chapter 3
- The Exorcism ✳: A deep healing for your lungs and your life—chapter 7
- The Red Suit: To prevent EIA—chapter 11
- The Golden Inhaler ✳: For immediate symptom relief—chapter 4
- Do unto Yourself: Be kind to yourself, generate joy—chapter 8

## Week Two
Continue to use: ssTUFF, Golden Inhaler, Red Suit, Do unto Yourself. Continue The Exorcism if you feel there is more to be accomplished, for two more weeks. Then, add the following:
- The Golden Bellows ✳: To strengthen and heal the lungs—chapter 4
- Taking a Weight off Your Chest ✳: To relieve and remove symptoms—chapter 4
- Create Your Own Top Twenty: Use music to express emotions and heal your life—chapter 7
- Turning Things Around: To disempower the Committee—chapter 7
- Create a Prayer Collage: To begin an asthma-free life—chapter 8

## Week Three
Continue to use: ssTUFF, Golden Inhaler, Red Suit, Do unto Yourself, Golden Bellows, Weight Off, Top Twenty. Then, add the following:
- The Singing Lung: To Undo or prevent breathing difficulties—chapter 7
- Clowning Around: To generate joy, lighten up, have fun—chapter 8

# THE 21-DAY HEALING PLAN FOR KIDS

## Week One

- The Exorcism ✳: A deep healing for your lungs and your life—chapter 7
- The FUN Collage: To create an image of an asthma-free life—chapter 10
- Box of Balloons: To generate a sense of freedom and relaxation—chapter 9

## Week Two

Continue to use: Box of Balloons and to work on the Collage. Then add the following:

- The Golden Inhaler ✳: To use in place of your regular inhaler—chapter 4
- The Rainbow Bridge ✳: To breathe freely. To prevent attacks—chapter 10
- Releasing Old Stuff: To get rid of old clutter and stuff—chapter 11

## Week Three

Continue to use: Box of Balloons (complete the 21 days), Golden Inhaler (as needed), and Rainbow Bridge. Work on the Collage if you like; the Collage can always change and grow. Then add the following:

- Create Your Own Imagery: Use Favorite Things list to make up imagery—chapter 10
- Pine Forest ✳: To stem an asthma symptom—chapter 10
- Do unto Others: Having FUN by being kind to others—chapter 8

## LAST WORDS

Whether you use one of these plans or create one of your own, think of this as an ongoing process—a mindbody prescription for an asthma-free life. This involves more than living without symptoms; it means being loving, productive, and personally empowered. Everything you've done here has shown you the way. Now it's time to take the leap. Don't be concerned about doing the plan perfectly or doing it all. Each part contains the whole, and doing even one exercise consistently may be enough to take you where you want to go. There's no right or wrong, pass or fail. When you place your trust in joy, freedom, and truth, the rest will inevitably follow; even your smallest effort can bear fruit. The following Complete Index may be used however suits you along the way.

## THE COMPLETE EXERCISE INDEX

### Chapter 3: Redefining Your Relationship with Asthma

SSTUFF: Exercise for Panic Prevention—To preclude panic

The Mindbody Asthma Questionnaire—To generate self-knowledge

### Chapter 4: Mind Medicine: Tapping into the Power of Imagination

Warm-Ups: A Brief Introduction to Imagery

* The Golden Inhaler—For immediate symptom relief
* The Golden Bellows—To strengthen and heal the lungs
* Taking a Weight off Your Chest—To relieve and remove symptoms

Seeing Is *Beliefing*—To create images of beliefs, feelings, and symptoms

## Chapter 5: The Road to Recovery: An Introduction to the **FUN** Program

The Freedom Exercise—To generate freedom and healing

Symptom Decoding—To understand the symptom's meaning

Road to Recovery—To energize and heal

## Chapter 6: Focus: The Art of Paying Attention

The Eye of the Beholder—To center yourself and to focus clearly

Transforming Symptoms by Watching—To stop judging and complaining

The Prison Cell—To focus on your willingness to be free

The Belief Inventory—To focus on your beliefs

Separating and Creating Space—To separate from beliefs, circumstances, events, and people

✳ You Are Not the Symptom—To separate from and release symptoms

Draw the Symptom—To define the symptom as a visible presence and separate from it

The Breathometer Exercise—To focus on when, why, where you hold your breath

Two of You—To cultivate your primary relationship, the one with yourself

## Chapter 7: Undo: Create the Healing Turn

Turning Things Around—To disempower your Committee; to Undo nocebos

✳ The Exorcism—A deep healing for your lungs and your life

Casting Out the Victimizer—To cast out, or Undo, Committee members

Hands of Time—To Undo a traumatic or distressing event of the past

Writing to Heal—To reduce or eliminate symptoms and need for medication

Decreating by Drawing—To eliminate the symptom

Create Your Own Dream Medicine—To Undo emotional difficulties, address symptoms, and heal life issues.

Create Your Own Top Twenty—Listen to music to express emotions and heal your life

✴ The Singing Lung—To Undo or prevent breathing difficulties; to have FUN

## Chapter 8: Now Act: Heal by Having Fun

Become Your Own Glyphologist—To read the signs for action in daily life

The Triple Mirror—To generate change, growth, and action

✴ Liberation from Slavery—To free yourself, emotionally and physically, from asthma

The Hero or Heroine—To eliminate obstacles (circumstantial, emotional, physical)

Clowning Around—To generate joy, have FUN, lighten up

Create a Prayer Collage—To release your old life (including the asthma) and begin anew

Do unto Others—To heal yourself through acts of kindness toward others

Do unto Yourself—To heal yourself through acts of kindness to yourself

The Golden Net—To manifest health, love, and joy in your life

## Chapter 9: Turning Work into Play: Mind Medicine to Empower Children

Box of Balloons—To generate a sense of freedom and relaxation; to relieve the asthma

The Family Tree—To correct family errors, including "genetic" illness

## Chapter 10: The **FUN** Guide for Kids

✴ The Pine Forest—To stem an asthma symptom

✴ The Rainbow Bridge—To breathe freely; to get rid of symptoms

✳ The Bubble Helmet—To protect yourself from bad air
Create Your Own Imagery—To make up your own healing
imagery
✳ The Sailboat—To feel free and happy
✳ Melting the Witch—To get rid of an asthma symptom
Making a FUN Collage—To create an asthma-free life

## Chapter 11: The Mindbody Way: Enviroment, Nutrition, and Exercise-Induced Asthma

Cleaning the Room—To use for environmental asthma prevention
Releasing Old Stuff—To release stuff from the past and free up
your life
The Red Suit—To generate energy and to prevent exercise-
induced asthma.

## Chapter 12: Asthma Free in 21 Days: Your Mindbody Plan for Healing

FUN Plan 1: A Healing Plan for Adults
FUN Plan 2: A Healing Plan for EIA
FUN Plan 3: A Healing Plan for Kids

# AFTERWORD

*Disease and health, like circumstances, are rooted in
thought. . . . Strong, pure and happy thoughts build up
the body in vigor and grace. The body is a delicate and
plastic instrument, which responds readily to the thoughts
by which it is impressed, and habits of thought will produce their own effects, good or bad, upon it.*

JAMES ALLEN, *As a Man Thinketh*

What James Allen wrote over a hundred years ago is as true and
relevant now as it was then. Yet for much of this century we have
ignored the connection between thought and health. So what has
made us return? What has moved us toward taking responsibility
for our health and healing, toward the realization that the healer
within is not a myth—that the mind is "real"? Could it be an evolution of character, a revival of spirit, or might it be our deep disappointment with the purely scientific approach to healing?

What an exquisite reversal we have begun since *mirth* and our
*beliefs* have become validated by the new scientific fields—slowly
transforming the popular perspective from disdain to reverence. For
centuries, we argued with ourselves: could it be possible that the
wisdom of the heart, intuition, dreams, images, glyphs, was as valuable as scientific thought? Even science admits that something is
going on, something that cannot be accounted for in the usual ways.
What was suspect for hundreds of years has been documented in
laboratories: fun generates health, laughter heals, joy strengthens
the heart and the lungs, and millions of us say—Aha! Eureka! As
though we had never heard this before.

But whether you rely on science to confirm it or use FUN to discover it for yourself, the truth remains constant: "There is no physician like cheerful thought."[1] For all of us who want to rid ourselves of asthma—or of any other disease—indeed, joy is the key. By remembering this we can all live asthma free, as we consciously choose life each moment, no matter what difficulties may come our way.

# NOTES

## Introduction

1. This statistic was issued by the Centers for Disease Control and Prevention in Atlanta for 1998, and shows that the number of asthma sufferers has more than doubled since 1980.
2. According to the *Journal of the American Medical Association* 280, no. 17 (1998).

## Chapter 1

1. The coloring process and imagery Kathryn Shafer used for healing the broken bones after her accident were based on *The Anatomy Coloring Book,* by Wynn Kabit and Lawrence Elson (New York: Addison-Wesley, 1993).

## Chapter 2

1. Carol W. Boyd, M.S., and Lillian B. Stone, B.S., eds., *Asthma Facts* (American Lung Association of Southeast Florida, 1999).
2. Betty Wray, *Taking Charge of Asthma* (New York: John Wiley & Sons, 1998), 141.
3. Maya Muir, "Beyond Steroids," *Alternative & Complementary Therapies* 4, no. 5 (1998): 305.
4. James Dalen, M.D., "'Conventional' and 'Unconventional' Medicine," *Archives of Internal Medicine* 158 (Nov. 4, 1998): 2179, 2180.
5. Katherine Gundling, M.D., "Why Did I Become an 'Allopath'?" *Archives of Internal Medicine* 158 (Nov. 4, 1998): 2185.
6. C. Kim and Y. S. Kwok, "Navajo Use of Native Healers," *Archives of Internal Medicine* 158 (Nov. 4, 1998): 2245–49.
7. Dalen, "'Conventional' and 'Unconventional' Medicine," 2179.
8. Erica Goode, "Your Mind May Ease What's Ailing You," *New York Times,* Apr. 18, 1999.
9. Denise Grady, "To Aid Doctors, AMA Journal Devotes Entire Issue to Alternative Medicine," *New York Times,* Nov. 11, 1998.

**Chapter 3**

1. David Mrazek, "Asthma, Stress, Allergies, and the Genes," in *Mind Body Medicine: How to Use Your Mind for Better Health*, ed. Daniel Goldman and Joel Gurin (New York: Consumer Reports Books, 1993), 196.
2. Sandra Blakeslee, "The Power of the Placebo Amazes Medical Experts," *New York Times*, Oct. 13, 1998.
3. Betty Wray, *Taking Charge of Asthma* (New York: John Wiley & Sons, 1998).
4. Larry Dossey, M.D., *Space, Time and Medicine* (Boston: New Sciences Library, 1982), 112.

**Chapter 4**

1. Gerald Epstein, *Healing Visualizations* (New York: Bantam, 1989), 35–36.
2. C. Caroselli and E. A. M. Barrett, "A Review of the Power as Knowing Participation in Change Literature," *Nursing Science Quarterly* 2, no. 1 (1998).
3. G. Epstein, E. A. M. Barrett, J. Halper, N. S. Seriff, K. Phillips, S. Lowenstein, "Alleviating Asthma with Mental Imagery: A Phenomenological Approach," *Alternative and Complementary Therapies* 3, no. 1 (Feb. 1997).
4. "The Golden Inhaler" is an exercise created by Dr. Gerald Epstein.
5. N. M. Edwards, L. Klauss, and F. Greenfield, "Effects of Group Imagery on Quality of Life and Functional Ability of Heart Failure Patients" (Columbia Presbyterian Medical Center, New York, 1998).
6. This exercise is adapted from Gerald N. Epstein, M.D., *Healing into Immortality: A New Spiritual Medicine of Healing Stories and Imagery* (New York: Bantam Books, 1994).
7. Holography is a process of lensless photography that was discovered in 1948 by Dennis Gabor. In holography, laser beams and mirrors are used to photograph an object, which is registered on a holographic plate as an energy pattern. When a laser beam is directed at this plate, a three-dimensional image reappears, as before, though somewhat less clearly. The process is outlined by Gerald Epstein, M.D., *Waking Dream Therapy* (Easthampton, NY: ACMI Press, 1992), 48.
8. Gerald Epstein, "Taking a Weight off Your Chest," *Alternative and Complementary Therapies* 3, no. 1 (Feb. 1997): 44.

9. The Committee was inspired by Richard D. Carson's concept of gremlin taming, from his book *Taming the Gremlin* (New York: HarperCollins, 1983).

10. John Carroll has since gone on to do this work with others. After healing himself, he discovered his gift as a spiritual healer and has since cultivated it. He works with people with many serious conditions, including cancer and asthma.

11. M. Merleau-Ponty, *Working Notes*, as quoted by James Hillman, *The Soul's Code: In Search of Character and Calling* (New York: Random House, 1996), xi.

12. The vertical and horizontal axis are illustrated in Valentin Tomberg's *Meditations on the Tarot* (New York: Amity House, 1985), 13.

13. Fran Greenfield, "Freedom to Heal" (1997), 13.

### Chapter 5

1. *American Heritage Dictionary*, 3d. ed.

2. Marilyn Ferguson, *The Aquarian Conspiracy* (Los Angeles: J. P. Tarcher, 1980).

3. Portia Nelson, *There's a Hole in My Sidewalk* (Hillsboro, OR: Beyond Words Publishing, 1993).

4. Virginia Satir, *Making Contact* (Berkeley, CA: Celestial Arts, 1976).

5. G. Epstein, *Healing Visualizations* (New York: Bantam, 1989), 72.

6. This statement was part of a private conversation between Larry Dossey and Michael Talbot, from *The Holographic Universe* (New York: HarperCollins, 1991), 89.

7. Moshe Mykoff, *The Empty Chair: Finding Hope and Joy: Timeless Wisdom from a Hasidic Master, Rebbe Nachman of Breslov* (Woodstock, VT: Jewish Lights Publishing, 1994), 110, 112.

### Chapter 6

1. Valentin Tomberg, *Meditations on the Tarot* (New York: Amity House, 1985), 8.

2. This is different from the Focusing process developed by Eugene Gendlin, in which you seek a "felt shift" and something is supposed to "happen" or "click into place." See his book, *Focusing* (New York: Bantam Books, 1981).

3. Marilyn Ferguson, *The Aquarian Conspiracy* (Los Angeles: J. P. Tarcher, 1980), 257, 69.

4. Joan Borysenko, *Minding the Body, Mending the Mind* (Reading, MA: Addison-Wesley, 1987), 20.

5. Sandra Blakeslee, "The Power of the Placebo," *New York Times*, Oct. 13, 1998.

6. Rachel Naomi Remen, *Kitchen Table Wisdom* (New York: Riverhead Books, 1996), 77.

7. Blakeslee, "Power of the Placebo."

8. Blakeslee, "Power of the Placebo."

9. The concept of separation and space as key elements for healing and freedom was shared with us by Dr. Gerald Epstein through his teachings and supervisions.

10. *Twelve Steps and Twelve Traditions* (New York: A. A. Grapevine and Alcoholics Anonymous World Services, 1981), 43.

11. James Hillman and Michael Ventura, *We've Had a Hundred Years of Psychotherapy—and the World's Getting Worse* (San Francisco: Harper-San Francisco, 1992).

12. Thich Nhat Hanh, *Being Peace* (Berkeley, CA: Parallex Press, 1987), 43.

13. Carl Stough, *Breathing: The Source of Life* (New York: Carl Stough Institute of Breathing Coordination, 1996).

14. Letha Hadady, *Asian Health Secrets* (New York: Crown Publishers, 1996), 101.

15. Fran Greenfield, "Freedom to Heal" (1997), 8.

16. "Two of You" is an exercise created by Joseph Shorr.

**Chapter 7**

1. *The I Ching or Book of Changes*, trans. Cary F. Baynes (Princeton: Princeton Univ. Press, 1980), 148, emphasis added.

2. Gerald Epstein, *Healing into Immortality* (New York: Bantam, 1994), 241.

3. Martin Rossman, "Imagery: Learning to Use the Mind's Eye," in *Mind Body Medicine: How to Use Your Mind for Better Health*, ed. Daniel Goldman and Joel Gurin (New York: Consumer Reports Books, 1993), 291–92.

4. Gerald Epstein, *Healing Visualizations* (New York: Bantam, 1989), 66, 67.

5. Epstein, *Healing Visualizations*, 66.

6. Gerald Epstein, "Hands of Time," in *Healing into Immortality* (New York: Bantam, 1994).

7. James Hillman, *The Soul's Code: In Search of Character and Calling* (New York: Random House, 1996), emphasis added.

8. Joshua Smyth, Arthur Stone, Alan Hurewitz, and Alan Kaell, "Effects of Writing About Stressful Experiences on Symptom Reduction in Patients with Asthma or Rheumatoid Arthritis," *Journal of the American Medical Association* 281, no. 14 (Apr. 14, 1999).

9. Strephon Kaplan Williams, *The Jungian-Senoi Dreamwork Manual* (Novato, CA: Journey Press, 1980), 176, emphasis added.

10. This dream reentry process was shared with the authors by Dr. Gerald Epstein.

11. Marilyn Ferguson, *The Aquarian Conspiracy* (Los Angeles: J. P. Tarcher, 1980), 166.

12. Don Campbell, *The Mozart Effect* (New York: Avon Books, 1997).

**Chapter 8**

1. Fran Greenfield, "Freedom to Heal" (1997), 9.

2. This observation was shared by Russell Mason in a conversation with Fran Greenfield.

3. Lawrence Hoffman, "The Clarity of Holy Names," *New York Jewish Week,* Dec. 25, 1998, 34.

4. "The Triple Mirror" is an exercise created by Madame Colette Aboulker-Muscat.

5. Greenfield, "Freedom to Heal," 32.

6. This list is based on the work of Dr. Bob Gibson and his model of the false self. Gibson's work is contained in an online catalog including books, tapes, videos, and transcripts at www.rhondell.com.

7. Greenfield, "Freedom to Heal," 55.

8. Marilyn Ferguson, *The Aquarian Conspiracy* (Los Angeles: J. P. Tarcher, 1980), 264.

9. In *Head First: The Biology of Hope* (New York: E. P. Dutton, 1989), 150–53, Norman Cousins includes lists of humorous books, audiocassettes, and videocassettes to use as action generators.

10. David Stout, "Doctor in Clown Suit Battles Ills of His Profession," *New York Times,* Dec. 15, 1998.

11. Stout, "Doctor in Clown Suit."

12. Reported by Claudia Dreifus, "A Mathematician at Play in the Fields of Space-Time," *New York Times,* Jan. 19, 1999.

13. Cousins, *Head First,* 127.

14. Proverbs 17:22.

15. Claudia Dreifus, "An Interview with Brooks and Reiner," *Modern Maturity,* March–April 1999, 32.

16. Jan Zeigler, "Immune System May Benefit from Ability to Laugh," *Journal of the National Cancer Institute* 87 (1994): 342–43.

17. Some of Kathy's favorite pieces for generating action include: "Every Breath You Take" by The Police; "Before You Accuse Me, Take a Look at Yourself" performed by Eric Clapton; "Exodus" by Bob Marley and the Wailers; "None of Us Are Free If One of Us Is Chained" by Ray Charles; "Angel" by Sarah McLachlan; and Beethoven's Seventh Symphony.

18. "The Golden Net" was shared with the authors by Dr. Gerald Epstein.

### Chapter 9

1. This exercise was shared with us by Dr. Gerald Epstein. Adults as well as children can use it.

2. American Academy of Allergy, Asthma, and Immunology Report, 1999.

3. Claudia Dowling, "Asthma Epidemic," *Life* (May 1997), 79.

4. American Academy of Allergy, Asthma, and Immunology Report, 1999.

5. D. A. Mrazek, M. D. Klinnert, P. Mrazek, and T. Macy, "Early Asthma Onset: Consideration of Parenting Issues," *Journal of the American Academy of Child and Adolescent Psychiatry* 30 (1991): 277–82.

6. Nina Bernstein, "38% Asthma Rate Found in Homeless Children," *New York Times,* May 5, 1999.

7. David Mrazek, "Asthma, Stress, Allergies, and the Genes," *Mind Body Medicine: How to Use Your Mind for Better Health,* ed. Daniel Goldman and Joel Gurin (New York: Consumer Reports Books, 1993), 199.

8. Valentin Tomberg, *Meditations on the Tarot* (New York: Amity House, 1985).

9. Eleanor Roosevelt, *You Learn by Living* (New York: Harper & Brothers, 1960), 4, emphasis added.

10. Neil Postman, *Technopoly: The Surrender of Culture to Technology* (New York: Vintage Books, 1993), 179.

11. Gerald Epstein, M.D., *Imaginetics* 1, no. 2 (July 1997).

12. This concept was inspired by information from Tomberg's *Meditations on the Tarot*.

13. Emily's images of the sun and the moon were inspired by an African folktale by Elphinstone Dayrell, *Why The Sun and the Moon Live in the Sky*.

### Chapter 10

1. "Pine Forest" is based on an exercise from Dr. Gerald Epstein's *Healing Visualizations* (New York: Bantam, 1989), 67.

### Chapter 11

1. "Cleaning the Room" is an exercise created by Dr. Gerald Epstein and contained in his book *Waking Dream Therapy* (New York: ACME Press, 1996).

2. *Diagnostic and Statistical Manual of Mental Disorders*, 4th ed. (Washington, DC: American Psychiatric Association, 1994), 44.

3. Robert Barkin et al., "The Dilemma of Drug Therapy for Multiple Personality Disorder," in *Treatment of Multiple Personality Disorder*, ed. Bennett G. Braun (Washington, DC: American Psychiatric Press, 1986), 107–32.

4. Gerald Epstein, *Healing Visualizations* (New York: Bantam, 1989), 200.

### Afterword

1. James Allen, *As a Man Thinketh* (Philadelphia: Running Press, 1989), 52.

# ABOUT THE AUTHORS

## Kathryn Shafer

Kathryn C. Shafer, Ph.D., LCSW, CAP, holds a master's degree from New York University and a doctorate from Barry University in Florida, both with concentrations in social work. For her doctoral research, Dr. Shafer developed an international substance abuse training curriculum for medical professionals in the former Soviet Union. Currently, she is an adjunct faculty member at several universities in Florida teaching undergraduate and graduate courses on psychology, substance abuse, social work practice, and social welfare history. Dr. Shafer works as a consultant to hospitals, substance abuse programs, and mental health centers on issues such as the clinical application of mindbody medicine, staff management, and program development.

Dr. Shafer first met Dr. Gerald Epstein in 1991 and quickly adopted his work in integrative medicine for her own healing and as the focus of the work in her clinical practice. She is a graduate of the American Institute for Mental Imagery, Dr. Epstein's school for postgraduate studies in New York City. She is also a graduate of the Mind-Body Institute at Harvard, under the direction of Dr. Herbert Benson. Dr. Shafer maintains a private practice in West Palm Beach, Florida, and in New York City called Limitless Potentials, where she counsels teens and adults with substance abuse, mental health, and medical problems. As an internationally certified play therapist, Dr. Shafer provides training for clinicians on the use of mental imagery for emotional and physical disorders in children, adolescents, and adults.

Dr. Shafer achieves remarkable success in her clinical practice using the FUN program to heal asthma, resolve emotional issues, stop addictive behavior, and increase health and stamina. She conducts workshops on these issues throughout the United States and abroad.

Dr. Shafer runs marathons asthma free without the use of medication.

She can be reached by e-mail at drshafer@gate.net.

## Fran Greenfield

For over twenty years, Fran Greenfield, M.A., has studied mindbody medicine, and has written extensively on this subject for publications that include the *New York Times*. Recognized as an expert in the field of imagination, she specializes in asthma, cancer, fertility, and personal growth. Her work empowers clients to transform physical and emotional difficulties into meaningful solutions that add joy to life.

At Columbia-Presbyterian Medical Center's Department of Complementary Medicine in New York City, she conducted research with heart-failure patients that demonstrated the measurable positive effects of mental imagery on their well-being. She has lectured on mindbody medicine at Columbia University's College of Physicians and Surgeons, and at the Medical Centers of New York's Beth Israel Hospital and Dartmouth College. In addition, Ms. Greenfield consults for SHARE, an organization for women with breast and ovarian cancer, and the Virginia Breast Cancer Foundation.

She holds a master's degree in counseling psychology and holistic studies, and has completed her postgraduate education at the American Institute for Mental Imagery. She is pursuing a doctoral degree in Traditions of Spiritual Healing, an exploration of ancient healing practices and their relevance for modern life.

Ms. Greenfield develops original therapeutic programs and trains health care professionals in techniques of integrative medicine. She also presents workshops for the public on the mindbody experience. She maintains private practices in New York City, on Long Island, and in Memphis, Tennessee.

She can be reached by e-mail at frangreenfield@earthlink.net.

# INDEX

Aboulker-Muscat, Madame Colette, 145, 171

action indicators: dreams as true, 164; false, 162–64; humor as, 166, 167–71. *See also* Now Act

actions: defining ourselves by, 173–77; do unto others, 175–76; do unto yourself, 176; music role in, 173

active listening, 148–49

acts of kindness, 174–77

Adams, Hunter D. ("Patch"), 167–68

African American asthmatics, 25

Alcoholics Anonymous, 106

Allen, James, 227

allergic irritants, 206–207

allergy trigger, 27–28

allopathic medicine: described, 31–32; medication side effects of, 33. *See also* conventional medicine

allopathy, 31–32, 34

alternative medicine asthma solutions, 2–3

American College of Allergy, Asthma, and Immunology, 39

*Anatomy of an Illness* (Cousins), 73, 167

angelic presence, 62, 65, 66–67

*Archives of Internal Medicine* (ed. by Dalen), 34

*As a Man Thinketh* (Allen), 227

*As Good as It Gets* (film), 191

asthma: defining, 24–25; demographics of, 25; exploring alternative approaches to, 2–3; failures of Western medicine for, 1–2;

redefining relationship with, 39–43; social/economic costs of, 1

asthma attacks: anatomy of Nora's, 38–43; signs and symptoms of, 25–26. *See also* asthma triggers; symptoms

asthma questionnaire, 43–45

asthma research: on childhood asthma risks, 184–85; on healing power of writing, 138–40; on imagery and need for medication, 54; on imagery used by seriously ill, 58–59; on power of imagery, 54–55

asthmatics: demographics of, 25; redefining relationship with asthma, 39–43; research study on imagery by, 54–55; varying severity suffered by, 24–25; Western medicine authoritarian model for, 2. *See also* children

asthma treatment: conventional medicine approach to, 31–35; meaningful phenomenon approach to, 30; traditional and natural approaches to, 33–35; using mental imagery techniques, 17–19, 22. *See also* mindbody perspective

asthma triggers: allergies as, 27–28; emotional stress as, 29–31; environmental, 28–31, 207–10; nutritional/food, 211–13; physical activity as, 29, 213–17; respiratory infection as, 29; work environment as, 28–29

attitude toward imagery, 50–51